# MANAGING PROJECTS IN HEALTH AND SOCIAL CARE

Change is a normal part of working life in public services and anyone who is a manager or professional leader can expect to have to lead projects that contribute to service development and improvement. *Managing Projects in Health and Social Care* is designed for anyone who is asked to manage a project but who lacks the experience or training to feel confident in this role. It shows, in detail, how to use project management techniques to ensure success, focussing on the key elements:

- budget
- time
- feasibility
- planning/scheduling
- implementation
- evaluation.

The book includes many examples to show how people have used project managment techniques effectively in health and care settings. There are clear explanations of how and when to use each technique and consideration of the differences between large, complex projects and smaller, less complicated ones. *Managing Projects in Health and Social Care* is a practical handbook for anyone who has responsibility for projects. It is a valuable resource for anyone who wants to be sure that their project will make a useful contribution to improvement of health and care services.

**Vivien Martin** is Senior Lecturer in the School of Health and Social Welfare, The Open University. She is co-author, with Euan Henderson, of *Managing in Health and Social Care*, also published by Routledge.

# MANAGING PROJECTS IN HEALTH AND SOCIAL CARE

Vivien Martin

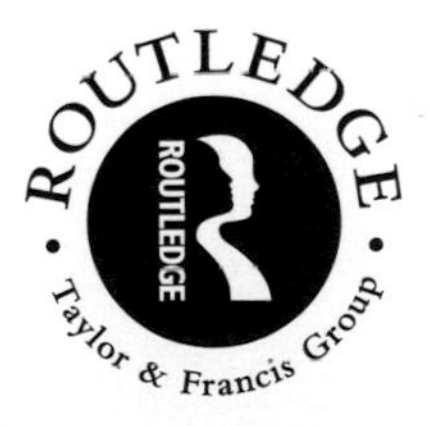


London and New York

First published 2002
by Routledge
11 New Fetter Lane, London EC4P 4EE

Simultaneously published in the USA and Canada
by Routledge
29 West 35th Street, New York, NY 10001

*Routledge is an imprint of the Taylor & Francis Group*



Designed and typeset in Futura and Sabon by Keystroke,
Jacaranda Lodge, Wolverhampton
Printed and bound in Great Britain by TJ International Ltd, Padstow, Cornwall



*British Library Cataloguing in Publication Data*
A catalogue record for this book is available from the British Library

*Library of Congress Cataloging in Publication Data*
A catalog record for this book has been requested

ISBN 0–415–27619–5 (HB)
ISBN 0–415–27620–9 (PB)

# CONTENTS

# ILLUSTRATIONS

## FIGURES



## TABLES

# EXAMPLES

# ACKNOWLEDGEMENTS

Some of the material in this book was developed during the production of the Open University Business School's Professional Diploma in Management. The contribution of the Programme team in developing this approach to the management of projects should be acknowledged. Acknowledgement should also be made to Helen Howard for her work on managing projects in the course 'Health and Social Services Management', developed by the Open Learning Foundation and the Open University. Thanks are also due to those who contributed directly and indirectly to the examples used in this book, in particular, Eddie Fisher and Stephen Oliver.

The Institute of Healthcare Managers have successfully encouraged first-line managers to develop projects as part of their Professional Certificate. Many of these projects have demonstrated the extent to which team leaders and first-line managers can contribute to the successful improvement of services. I hope that this book will provide practical support and increase the confidence of those who give their energy and commitment to service development.

Figure 2.2 'The classic six-stage project management model' is reproduced from *Project Skills* (1988) by Sam Elbeik and Mark Thomas. Reprinted by permission of Butterworth-Heinemann.

Vivien Martin, 2001

# INTRODUCTION

This book will provide you with a practical approach to managing a project in a health or care setting. People who have leadership or functional responsibilities are increasingly expected to manage projects as part of their day-to-day work. Few receive special training to help them to take on this task, although it is very different from professional, clinical or functional roles in health and social care. If you are one of these people, help is at hand!

This book provides a practical introduction to management of projects and will be a useful handbook for help in any future projects you find yourself invited to manage. It focuses on projects that might be carried out by team leaders, and first-line and operational managers, but will also be attractive to more senior people who are managing projects for the first time. Each chapter discusses an aspect of project management and illustrates the discussion with examples drawn from health and care settings. Techniques are described and applied to examples and there are activities to encourage you to try out different approaches. Further references are provided for those managing larger or more substantial and long-term projects. There are also references to sources of information about leadership, consultative management style, 'change-management' approaches and influencing skills, without which the management of any project can run into difficulties.

Projects are usually intended to contribute to development and change within an organisation or service area. The context of health and social care is complex, with many different interests to consider. The patients or users of health and social care services are often vulnerable during their contact with the service and change can be disruptive to service users and to staff. It is important that projects improve the service without reducing the quality offered to service users or putting additional strain on staff who already work within limited resources. Successful management of a project is quite a balancing act and can only be learnt through experience and reflection on experience, supported by thoughtful consideration of the ideas, processes and techniques that have become recognised as the expertise of project management.

The opportunity to take responsibility for a project offers personal and career development as well as the opportunity to contribute to achieving a worthwhile change.

## HOW TO USE THIS BOOK

The chapters are arranged in roughly the order of things that you need to consider when managing a project. Unfortunately, however, projects do not often progress neatly through one logical stage after another. If you are managing a project for the first time you might find it useful to glance through the overview of chapters and note the issues that are raised so that you can plan how to make best use of the book to support your own learning needs.

Projects come in many different shapes and sizes and some of the techniques and processes described here will seem unnecessarily complicated for small projects. In some cases, the processes can be reduced or carried out more informally when a project is not too large or complicated, but beware of missing out essential basic thinking. The chapter on scoping a project and that about developing the evidence base focus on making sure that the project has a clear and appropriate aim and enough support to achieve its purpose. Many projects founder because they are set up quickly to address issues that people feel are very urgent and the urge to take action means that the ideas are not fully considered. Rushing the initial thinking can result in failure to achieve objectives and even more delay.

There is more scope for taking a simpler approach in the planning and implementation stages. Planning is not a one-off activity but more like a continuous cycle of plan, do, review and plan again. With a small team and in a setting where people are comfortable with flexible working, the sharing and sequencing of tasks might be quickly agreed. If you are managing a project that does not need some of the techniques that are offered in these chapters then don't use them – there is no one 'right' way to manage or lead a project. Each project is different and you need to develop the knowledge and flexibility to be able to match your management approach to each individual project. It helps to have a broad general knowledge about a variety of approaches so that you can be selective and make an appropriate choice.

You might like to think of the book as support for your personal approach when you take responsibility for a project. Consult the book to give you confidence that you have thought through the main issues. Use it to prepare for important meetings. Check the relevant chapters as you move through the stages of the project. Take the opportunities for learning and self-development offered by participation in a project and keep the book on your shelf for the next time. Successful project managers are always in demand!

Many people following courses leading to qualifications will have to complete a work-based project as part of their study. This is an opportunity to make a contribution to your work area as well as to progress your own development. This book is written to support the practical roles of a person leading or managing a project in a health or care workplace, but the models, techniques, processes and concepts introduced are those considered in professional and management courses of study. There are few references in the text, but a section at the end of the book offers suggestions for further reading and other resources for those who want to study this area of management in more detail.

## OVERVIEW OF CHAPTERS

*Chapter 1 – What is a project?* – Some characteristics of projects in health and care services are discussed. This leads to the importance of clarifying the purpose and setting clear aims and objectives. Some of the features that are common to any project are identified and their importance discussed. The chapter concludes with a consideration of the main purpose of a project, the outcomes that are to be achieved.

*Chapter 2 – Scoping the project* – takes you through several ways of identifying where the boundaries to a project lie. Two of the most commonly used models of project management are introduced and used to help to clarify the choices to be made.

*Chapter 3 – Making evidence-based decisions* – It is often tempting to move straight into planning a project once an idea has been enthusiastically shared. This chapter encourages you to check, from a number of different perspectives, whether there is any evidence to support the idea. The focus is on questioning whether the project is worth doing and whether it will be able to achieve what it is intended to do. Option appraisal is discussed and the potential benefits of carrying out a pilot study are considered.

*Chapter 4 – Defining the project* – The focus here is on developing a detailed project brief that will be signed by the person responsible for funding the project and supported by all of the key stakeholders in the project.

*Chapter 5 – Managing risk* – This offers an approach to management of risk and contingency planning. Risk is inevitable in a project and it would be impossible to achieve anything without exposing ourselves to some degree of risk. The chapter covers risk assessment and impact analysis and suggests some strategies for dealing with risk.

*Chapter 6 – Outline planning* – Addresses the question of, Where do I start? Some straightforward approaches to developing a project plan are explained to help you to identify exactly what the project must produce.

*Chapter 7 – Estimating time and costs* – Once the outline plans have been developed, estimates will be needed for the costs of the activities that contribute to the project and for the time that each activity will take. More information is needed to make these estimates and this chapter introduces a structured approach to planning the work of a project so that these estimates can be made with some confidence.

*Chapter 8 – Scheduling* – covers the timing and sequence of activities in the project. The sequence is very important when one task must be completed before another begins. The time that each task will take needs to be estimated before the length of the project can be confirmed and this overall time will depend on the extent to which tasks and activities have to be delayed until others are completed. Some basic techniques are introduced that will help you to make these calculations.

*Chapter 9 – Implementing the project* – This is the exciting stage in a project when the plans begin to be enacted. The focus moves to managing action and ensuring that the project team or teams can start work and understand what is needed. The project manager needs also to consider how to secure personal support when it is needed and how to retain an overview while responding to the inevitable detail of the day-to-day tasks.

*Chapter 10 – Monitoring and control* – Monitoring entails the collection of information about the progress of activities during the implementation phase of a project. It is essential to monitor if you are to be able to control progress on the project. The monitoring information can be reviewed against the plan to show whether everything is proceeding according to the plan. If not, the project manager can bring the project back into control by taking action to recover the balance of time, cost and quality.

*Chapter 11 – Communications* – focuses on the need for effective communications in a project and the things that a project manager can do to provide appropriate systems. Much of the communication in a project is in connection with sharing information. Management of the flow of information is considered alongside a reminder of the responsibility of the project manager in ensuring that confidentialities are respected.

*Chapter 12 – Leadership and teamworking* – After some comment on the nature of leadership in health and social care, this chapter focuses on leadership issues in a project. Leadership and teamworking are closely linked and motivation is also considered.

*Chapter 13 – Managing performance* – One of the things that a project manager can do in the early stages of a project is to prepare for good performance. It is much easier to manage performance to ensure that the project is successful if the performance requirements have been made specific and the staff have been adequately prepared. If the worst happens and a manager has to deal with poor performance it is essential to have policies and procedures in place to ensure that the actions taken are legal and fair to the individuals concerned.

*Chapter 14 – Completing the project* – The implementation of a project ends with completion but there are often a number of outcomes with elements that have to be handed over to the project sponsor. There are choices about how these things are delivered. There are also a number of steps to take in ensuring that a project is closed properly so that any remaining resources are accounted for and all of the contractual relationships have been concluded.

*Chapter 15 – Evaluating the project* – Most projects end with an evaluation and it often falls to the project manager to design and plan the process. This chapter outlines the process and ends with some consideration of the issues that may arise in presenting a report.

*Chapter 16 – Reporting the project* – This chapter deals with two areas that often worry project managers: how to develop a full written report and how to make an oral presentation. Different types of reports are appropriate for different types of audience, so different types of decision need to be made when preparing either a written or oral report.

*Chapter 17 – Learning from the project* – Most projects will have aspects that go well and others that do not go so well. There is always a lot that can be learnt but much of the learning will be lost if care is not taken to ensure that it is captured. There is also considerable potential for personal learning and for management development during a project.

The book concludes with a brief note about further reading that may be helpful for anyone managing a project in health or social care.

CHAPTER 1

# WHAT IS A PROJECT?

Many people in different roles in health and care organisations find themselves working on projects from time to time and will sometimes be asked to lead or manage a project. Sometimes we are asked to join a project team as part of our workload and sometimes we are seconded to work exclusively on a project for a defined period of time. Some people are appointed to fixed-term jobs that are entirely concerned with work on one specific project. So what is a project? We use the word 'project' to describe something that is not part of ordinary day-to-day work. It also indicates something that is purposeful and distinct in character. In this chapter we shall consider how to distinguish a project from other work and some of the characteristics of projects in health and care settings. We shall also outline some of the factors that contribute to successful completion of projects.

## PROJECTS IN HEALTH AND CARE SERVICES

Health and care services are often in the public spotlight because they are so central to the well-being of communities. Unfortunately there is often more excited interest when there is a tragic failure of services than when things go well. Any breakdown in services leads to a call for improvement. There is always pressure to improve services, often in response to perceived failings. Pressure to change public services also comes from developments in government policy in attempts to meet public expectations of high-quality services.

People often say that change is the only constant in organisational life. This is probably true of your experience if you work in health or care services. People who have been in such work for a number of years will have experienced frequent changes in the way that provision is structured and funded and in the ways in which we deliver health and care services to service users. Such change is not limited to public services dependent on government funding. As public expectations change, all service providers are challenged to meet new and differing expectations. Voluntary and private health and care organisations are dependent on being regarded as good value to those who pay for their services.

Projects at work can consist of many different types. Some may be short-term, for example organising a special event, making a major purchase or moving an office. Or they may be bigger, longer and involve more people, for example if the project involves developing a new service or a new function or moving a service area to a new location. The project may be expected to deliver an improvement to service provision. It may be expected to deliver financial benefits to the organisation in some way. In the public sector, projects are normally expected to lead to social, economic and political outcomes.

Projects contribute to the management of change. You might reasonably think that there is no point in carrying out a project if it does not result in a change. However:

- change management usually refers to substantial organisational change that might include many different types of change in many different areas of work;
- project management usually refers to one specific aspect of the change.

Therefore, projects are often distinct elements in wider organisational change.

**Example 1.1 – A project as part of change management**

A large hospital with acute and emergency services was merging with a smaller community healthcare organisation that offered a range of clinical and professional services in local surgeries and through home visits to patients. The development of the new merged organisation was a long and complex process, but a number of projects were identified that contributed to the change process. These included:

- development of new personnel policies;
- relocation of Directorate offices;
- disposal of surplus estates;
- development and implementation of financial systems for the new organisation;
- development and implementation of new management information system.

Many other changes were less well defined, for example team building among the new teams of directors, managers, clinical and professional leaders and functional teams.

# FEATURES OF A PROJECT

We normally use the term 'project' in quite a precise way although it can encompass many different types of activity. It can refer to a short personal project, for example planning and holding a special celebration. It can also refer to a major construction, for example a project to build a new hospital. All projects are different but they do have certain features in common. A project:

- has a clear purpose that can be achieved in a limited time;
- has a clear end when the outcome has been achieved;
- is resourced to achieve specific outcomes;
- has someone acting as a sponsor or commissioner who expects the outcomes to be delivered on time;
- is a one-off activity and would not normally be repeated.

As in any activity within an organisation, there are constraints which limit the process in various ways. For example, policies and procedures may constrain the ways in which things are done. The outcomes that are required may be defined very precisely and measures may be put in place to ensure that the outcomes conform to the specified requirements. Once a project has been defined, it is possible to estimate the resources that will be needed to achieve the desired outcomes within the desired time. A project is usually expected to achieve outcomes that will be required only once and so projects are not normally repeated. Even if a pilot project is set up to try out an idea, the outcome from the pilot should achieve what was required without the need to conduct another pilot project (unless different ideas are subsequently to be explored). Working on a project is not like ongoing everyday work processes unless all of your work is focused through project working.

## ACTIVITY 1.1

*Allow two minutes.*

Which of the following activities would you consider to be projects?

| | | *Yes* | *No* |
|---|---|---|---|
| (a) | Developing a new, documented induction procedure | ❐ | ❐ |
| (b) | Establishing a jointly agreed protocol to review the quality provided by a new cleaning service. | ❐ | ❐ |
| (c) | Maintaining client records for an outpatients service. | ❐ | ❐ |
| (d) | Managing staff rotas. | ❐ | ❐ |
| (e) | Transferring client records from a card file to a new computer system. | ❐ | ❐ |
| (f) | Setting up a management information system | ❐ | ❐ |

We would say that (a), (b) and (e) come within our definition of a project, whereas (c) and (d) are routine activities and are therefore not projects. In the case of (f) it is important to distinguish between the development of a management information system (which might benefit from a project management approach) and the subsequent process of ensuring that appropriate data are entered into the system and used for management, which is part of everyday activity.

---

Managing or leading a project is different from taking such a role in everyday work simply because of the limited nature of a project. There is a time limit that restricts the length of time that anyone in the project team will be in that role. There is a limit to the type of work that an individual is expected to contribute to the project. Some members of a project team may be selected to bring expertise in their professional or clinical field and others will be selected for other reasons. For example, an experienced nurse might be asked to lead a project team whose task is to develop an induction process and documentation not because of her or his expertise in nursing but because that person has demonstrated leadership in day-to-day work.

**Example 1.2 – The multidisciplinary mental health team**

A team was established in a London borough as part of an initiative intended to improve joint working across the different services contributing to mental health provision. The team included managers, doctors, clinical psychologists, counsellors and special needs teachers. At first many of the participants were sceptical about whether the team would be able to achieve anything, as the membership was so diverse. As time developed, the team began to understand how it could make a useful contribution by drawing on the range of different expertise brought by the participants. One of the first successes was the production of a local directory of services that identified contacts in public, private and voluntary services in the area. Many team members said that they found it much easier to work together when they had agreed a clear target, although in the early meetings the different perspectives taken from each specialism caused considerable friction. Some people thought a lot of time was wasted while others struggled to understand why they appeared to be putting obstacles in the way. However, once there was a project under way that could only work when each source of specialist knowledge was included, the benefits of joint working were accepted and welcomed.

## AIMS

It is often said that aims describe the ultimate goal, the purpose of the project, while objectives describe the steps that are necessary to achieve that goal. If you ask, 'What is the purpose of the project?' this will help to identify the overall aims. The aims can also be described as the vision. In some ways, using the word 'vision' is helpful as it implies having a picture of success. Aims can encompass values alongside purpose, which is helpful as they can describe the outcome in terms of how it should be achieved. They can also identify any important aspects of the outcome that relate to the values of the service. Aims can express a vision and describe a purpose, but clear objectives provide the details that describe how the aim will be achieved.

## SETTING CLEAR OBJECTIVES

It is very important to set clear objectives because these describe exactly what you are aiming to achieve and will provide the only way in which you will know whether you have succeeded or not. It is often easy to agree the broad goals of the project, but these need to be translated into objectives if they are to be used to plan the project and to guide the assessment of whether the project has achieved what was intended.

Objectives are clear when they define what is to be achieved, say when it is to be completed and explain how everyone will know that the objective has been achieved. Many people use the word SMART to remind themselves of the areas to consider when setting clear objectives:

- Specific – clearly defined with completion criteria;
- Measurable – you will know when they have been achieved;
- Achievable – within the current environment and with the skills that are available;
- Realistic – not trying to achieve the impossible;
- Timebound – limited by a completion date.

If you write objectives that include all of these aspects you will have described what has to be done to achieve the objective. This makes objectives a very useful tool in a planning process. However, as planning often has to be revisited as events unfold, you will also find that you have to revisit objectives and, maybe, revise them as you progress through the project. This is when aims can be very helpful in reminding everyone of the intentions and purpose.

**Example 1.3 – A clear objective**

An objective for a refurbishment project might be stated as: 'To replace the flooring in the entrance area'.

This objective meets some of the criteria of a SMART objective, but not others. It is reasonably specific, assuming that it is clear where the floor of the entrance area finishes, perhaps where it meets other types of flooring. However, it does not give any information about the type of flooring. Presumably the completion criteria would have aspects of quality, time-scale and cost which also are not mentioned here. How shall we know when the objective has been completed successfully? We might know when the flooring has been replaced but we won't know how successful the project has been unless we know more about whether it was achieved within the budget and the extent of disruption allowed in the environment and whether it was finished on time. A more SMART objective could be written as:

> To replace the flooring in the entrance area with hard-wearing carpet tiles that will be fitted in sections to reduce disruption and will be completed by September 30th within a budget of £1,000.

It is now clear that success can be measured by quality of carpet tiles, time-scale and budget and also in terms of the degree of reducing disruption during the process of replacing the flooring.

There will usually be a number of objectives to complete in order to achieve the goals of a project. These objectives can be grouped into clusters that lead to completion of different parts of the project.

Objectives are important in two ways in a project:

- they identify exactly what has to be done, and
- they allow you to establish whether or not each objective has been achieved.

The objectives that you set in the early stages of the project provide a framework for the final evaluation. They also provide information that will help you to monitor the progress of the project so that it can be controlled and managed.

## KEY DIMENSIONS OF A PROJECT

There are three key dimensions to a project:

- budget
- time
- quality

and these have to be balanced to manage a project successfully. A successfully completed project would finish on time, within the estimated budget and having achieved all of the quality requirements. These three dimensions of budget, time and quality are often regarded as the aspects of a project that must be kept in an appropriate balance if the project is to achieve a successful outcome. The job of the person leading or managing the project is to keep a balance that enables all of these dimensions to be managed effectively (Figure 1.1).

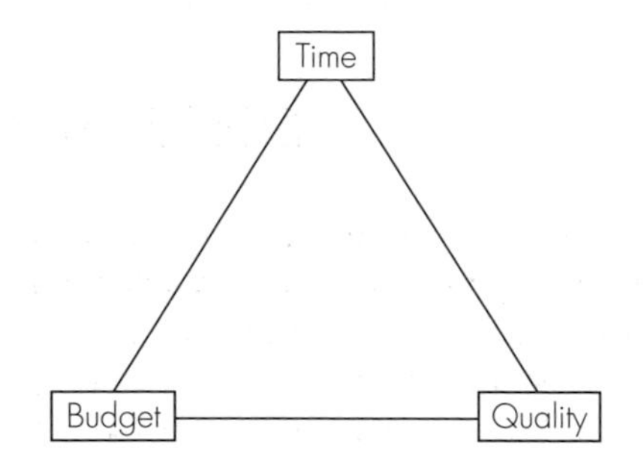


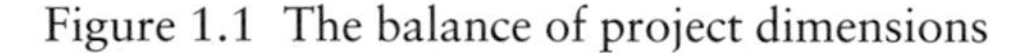

Figure 1.1 The balance of project dimensions

These dimensions are in tension with each other and any action focused on one of the dimensions will impact on both of the others. For example, if a reduction is made in the budget, there might be an impact on the time-scale if fewer people are available to carry out the activities or there might be an impact on the quality of the outcomes if the activities are rushed. These dimensions are useful to keep in mind throughout the progress of a project because actions and decisions will often impact on one or another of these dimensions and upset the balance. If the balance is upset, the danger is that the project will fail to meet the expectations of keeping within the agreed budget, finishing by the target date or producing outcomes of the quality required.

**Example 1.4 – An unbalanced project**

A project was set up within a hospital to improve the area in which out-patients waited. A budget was agreed to cover decoration of the walls, a new carpet and new seating. The work started but soon ran into problems as the workmen who were preparing the walls found that the ceiling was dangerously unstable and that sections of it would have to be replaced. The project manager gained agreement to increase the budget to allow for this additional work. However, the work on the ceiling delayed completion of the wall decorations. This caused problems in timing, because the carpet had been ordered so that it could be fitted as soon as the walls were completed. The delay to carpet fitting had an impact on the delivery of the new furniture, which also had to be delayed. Decorators worked in screened-off parts of the room and the waiting space for the patients was considerably reduced. This reduced the quality of service provided for these patients and their relatives, although the long-term intentions were to improve the quality of the area. The manager of this project had to frequently switch his attention from budget to time and then to quality, considering the impact on each of these dimensions as the project progressed.

## PEOPLE IN PROJECTS

Although the model of dimensions helps us to keep an overview of projects, another crucial dimension to keep in mind is the involvement of people in projects. People commission and sponsor projects, agree to provide resources, support or challenge projects and give their energy and intelligence to carry out projects. People take roles in delivering projects as leaders, managers and team members and also influence projects as sponsors, stakeholders, mentors, coaches, expert advisers and in other roles. With so many people involved, projects are strongly influenced by how these people feel and talk about the project and how they behave in relation to the project.

People are central to every aspect of a project.

**Example 1.5 – A project sensitive to people**

A consultancy service was commissioned by a Regional Health Office to provide a development programme for senior managers. There was considerable interest in what would be provided and who would be presenting the programme because many people thought that participation in it would influence promotion decisions. The consultants developing the programme recognised that the project was very sensitive in terms of involvement. Most sensitive decisions would involve the people selected to be participants in the programme. However, there were also other roles to consider. These included selection of the people who presented elements of the programme and people who were involved as line managers and mentors. It was also crucial to develop good relationships with people who acted as evaluators for the commissioners. As the ultimate purpose of the project was to improve services to service users, some involvement from users was important. There was also interest from the press and from professional and accreditation bodies.

This project managed the extensive range of interests by designing each aspect of the project in a way that involved those with particular interests and concerns. This included carrying out more than fifty interviews with directors as part of the development of a competence framework for senior managers aspiring to directorships. Senior managers and directors were also trained to make the selection decisions. This emphasised that the development programme was 'owned' by those who would make promotion decisions.

## OUTCOMES AND MULTIPLE OUTCOMES

A project is usually intended to achieve at least one distinct outcome. For example, a project to develop and test an induction manual should do exactly that. The project brief should identify all of the outputs that will be required to ensure that the project is 'signed off' as successful.

It is possible, however, to build in other outcomes that add value to the activity. One obvious opportunity is to use the project to enable personal development for those carrying out the various tasks. Alongside staff development, there might be an opportunity for a team to work together to develop their teamworking approach, although project teams are usually temporary and assembled only to complete the project. Projects are often used as part of individual staff development to give experience of planning, managing and leading a team. If you are able to demonstrate that you have successful experience in managing a project, it can contribute to your promotion prospects. Also, projects are often used as vehicles for learning when people are studying for qualifications.

Projects offer rich opportunities for staff development. These include opportunities to plan and manage the project, to liaise with people at different levels within the organisation and to carry out and report on the progress of numerous tasks. Any project can be viewed as a set of specific tasks and activities, each of which demands skills and experience to be performed well, but also offers the opportunity for someone to gain the necessary skills and experience if suitable training or coaching is provided. This last point is crucial and carries implications for all aspects of the project. If the project is to be used as a training ground, the necessary support must be built into the planning and the resourcing if the outcomes are to be expected on time, within the agreed budget and to the desired quality.

Projects are often required as part of educational courses because they give an opportunity for students to demonstrate that they can apply the course concepts and ideas in an integrated way in a real situation. It is also usually a requirement that the students should demonstrate that they can review the results and provide a critical evaluation of what was achieved and what was learnt from the project.

## ACHIEVING OUTCOMES

Unfortunately, projects do not always achieve all of their intended outcomes. The key dimensions of a project (budget, time and quality) suggest where problems might arise:

- the project might run over budget (or have to stop because of lack of funding before the objectives are achieved);
- it might take much longer to achieve the objectives than had been estimated (or might have to stop early because time runs out);
- it might be completed within the time and budget but not be of sufficiently high quality (and so be of less value than intended).

If there were failures in any of these dimensions there would be considerable waste of time, money and effort. The achievement would be considerably less than had been expected. People will be disappointed and there might be loss of reputation for those who are perceived to have been responsible for the failure.

There are many factors that contribute to completion of a project, and, therefore, many things that can contribute to success.

---

### ACTIVITY 1.2

*Allow 5 minutes.*

From your experience, list the most important factors that have contributed to the success of any projects in which you have been involved. Which three factors would you rank as most important?

| *Factor* | *Rank* |
| --- | --- |
| ________________ | ________________ |
| ________________ | ________________ |
| ________________ | ________________ |
| ________________ | ________________ |
| ________________ | ________________ |
| ________________ | ________________ |
| ________________ | ________________ |

You might have identified that it is very important to have enough time to complete the necessary tasks. You may even have been involved in a project that suddenly became urgent and everything was required more quickly than had been originally planned. Also, many people will have experience of being short of resources in health and care settings. If you have been involved in projects where you were not sure what was required or where the requirements seemed to keep changing, you will be aware of the need for clear objectives and for a shared understanding of those objectives.

---

Planning is very important in all stages of a project. You need to have clear objectives so that everyone can understand what you are trying to achieve. Planning is necessary to set out the steps that must be taken to achieve the objectives. Once activities begin, you need to check that everything is progressing according to the plan and to be prepared to take action to correct things if there are delays or difficulties. These planning, monitoring and control activities are the main responsibilities of the person managing the project. There are also leadership responsibilities. Good communications and interpersonal relationships are crucial to the ways in which people work together.

It is fortunate that quite a lot is known about how to manage projects successfully. If you are new to the roles of managing and leading projects you will find that careful preparation can help you to deliver successful outcomes.

CHAPTER 2

# SCOPING THE PROJECT

A project can be distinguished from the complexity of change in organisations because it is limited by boundaries and focused on a particular issue or set of issues. All projects are different because they are intended to achieve something specific in a setting that is in constant change. A project is temporary but it is intended to create a new product or service. The scoping stage of a project is about identifying the size and shape of the project and describing it in a way that helps everyone concerned to understand the intentions. Scoping is essentially about deciding what is 'in' the project and what is 'outside' the scope of the project.

Health and social care services are always under pressure to change, to meet increasingly demanding expectations of government policies and service users. On a local level, individual patients and service users want services that meet individual needs. Any project that aims to improve an aspect of health and social care provision will have to be understood from many different perspectives in a complex setting. Moreover, everyone in the setting who should normally be included in shaping and focusing the project is likely to be very busy and concerned with meeting immediate demands. This may make it difficult to gain their attention unless the project seems to offer benefits that are worth trying to achieve.

It is often tempting to try to include the priorities of all of the most influential people within a project, so that their support may be gained. Although there may be opportunities to address several organisational priorities within a project, it is usually dangerous to try to achieve too many diverse objectives. There is a danger of not achieving the main purpose if the project tries to bend in too many different directions. Scoping the project should enable you to identify exactly what work should be included to achieve the intended outcome successfully. The process will also clarify what should not be seen as part of the project but might be considered for a different project or perhaps as an area for continuous improvement.

If you do not spend time scoping the project a number of things can go wrong. For example:

- goals and objectives may be unclear, causing difficulties in deciding how they might be achieved;
- people might waste time and energy trying to achieve more than is realistic;
- people may try to solve the wrong problem;
- the objectives may contain contradictory elements that make them impossible to achieve.

In order to scope the project you will need to gain an overview of it. A number of models can be used to gain an overview of a project. Some of these emphasise the sequence of stages through which a project will normally progress. Others propose key areas that must be managed carefully if the project is to be successful. To some extent, the different models provide different views of a project and you can use them to check that you have thought through all of the main aspects.

We will use the examples in this chapter to try out the models and to consider how much each might help us to 'scope' a project.

**Example 2.1 – A project to scope**

Our example is a project that aims to improve the rehabilitation of elderly people into the community after health care treatment in a hospital. The project has arisen because the hospital is facing increasing demand for beds and frequently is unable to accommodate local patients. There is a general perception that a number of beds are being occupied by elderly people who could go home if there was enough help to support them to regain previously independent lives. The proposed project is to improve the rehabilitation arrangements in order to avoid beds being 'blocked' by elderly patients who no longer need to be treated in a hospital bed.

Chris is a nurse who works on a ward for elderly people and has been asked to manage the project. Chris has been asked to scope the project for a meeting next week. Chris starts by considering whether the Project Life Cycle model would help the meeting to gain an overview of the project.

# THE LIFE OF A PROJECT

The project life-cycle model (Figure 2.1) describes the different phases that a project normally passes through as it progresses to a conclusion. The model is based on the idea that, although all projects are different, they all progress through similar phases. Each phase can be identified because it completes a phase of the project. For example, the first phase is called project definition and it is completed when the project has been thoroughly defined so that a description called the project brief has been written and agreed.

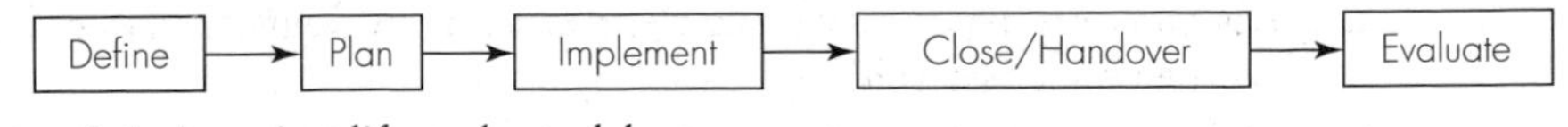


Figure 2.1 A project life-cycle model

In this model there are five phases:

- Phase 1 – Project definition. This is completed when the project brief has been written and agreed.
- Phase 2 – Planning. This includes all of the elements that make up the project plan.
- Phase 3 – Implementation. This includes all of the activities and tasks that achieve the project outcomes.
- Phase 4 – Closure. This includes all of the activities and tasks that ensure that the project is completely finished.
- Phase 5 – Evaluation. This may include evaluation of the processes used in the project and of the outcomes achieved.

The idea of a life cycle considers that a project has a life. This implies a sequence of phases, including birth, growth, maturity, ageing and death. We talk of the 'life' of a project, accepting that it exists for a limited time. During that time we expect it to grow and achieve its outcomes and then to close. The project's 'history' develops as the team or successive teams and the individuals who contribute make decisions and carry out activities. The project history influences each successive phase since decisions and actions both provide foundations and limit the possibilities that follow. We might also be sorry when a project ends, even if it has achieved all of its aims, because the end signals the end of the collaborative work for those who contributed.

**Example 2.2 – Using the project life-cycle model**

Chris made some quick notes to try out the project life-cycle model as a way of providing an overview of the rehabilitation project. Here are the notes:

*Phase 1 – Project definition*
The project is about the rehabilitation of elderly people after hospital treatment. They need to be helped back to lives in their own homes and communities. The hospital needs to use their beds once their treatment is complete. How do we turn this into a project brief? Who needs to agree the brief?

*Phase 2 – Planning*
We need to decide what has to be done to improve rehabilitation. That will certainly include more people than those in the hospital – perhaps social workers or residential care managers. In the hospital we'll have to include medical staff as well as nurses and physiotherapy and probably occupational

therapy professionals. There is a lot to do in discussing the situation before we can plan what to do about it. It will take ages to get everyone together.

*Phase 3 – Implementation*
We can't start doing things until we have decided what to do – so implementation will have to wait until after consultations and decisions about possible actions. I suppose this means that nothing will happen very quickly.

*Phase 4 – Closure*
I'm not sure how this project will close – perhaps we'll design a new protocol or set of processes that we'll all agree to follow. We all think we'll need to have better communications with people in other services so we'll need some way of agreeing how to work together and whose budget will cover what areas of work. I hope we'll be able to work together afterwards as a multi-professional team and not have to finish working together just because the project has finished.

*Phase 5 – Evaluation*
We'll need to evaluate whether we've made a difference. It's not just about counting beds, but more about whether we can help the patients get back to normal life. That might be difficult to evaluate, but it has to be the most important aspect of the project. We might also think about evaluating how we've worked together as a multiprofessional project team – that would be useful for future working.

The life-cycle model has helped to identify some of the areas that will need consideration, especially the amount of time that will be needed to involve others in discussions. Thinking about the phases has helped to show that the project definition phase will have to be carried out thoroughly with all those involved in the problem area before it is clear where the problems lie or where improvement might be made.

---

## ACTIVITY 2.1

What do you think Chris still needs to consider in scoping this project?

________________________________________

________________________________________

________________________________________

________________________________________

________________________________________

The purpose of the project will have to be much clearer before it is possible to begin the planning phase. It will also be important to identify a budget and a time-scale so that the project can be managed effectively.

This project will need a lot of different people to be involved in defining what the problems really are and understanding whether these are problems in how different services work together or perhaps problems that arise because there are no services that would be appropriately involved. It almost sounds as though there should be a project to decide whether there should be a further project – the scoping phase might be a project in itself.

The ownership of this project might be a problem. Chris needs to think a lot more about the nature of the problem and the objectives of the project. Although the hospital have identified it from the perspective of beds being occupied by older people who could be back in their own homes with a little help, this might not be how either the elderly patients or the social and community services see the issues. This project might be more about how to work across the relevant service areas to develop care plans for older people at the point where they are identified as in need of hospital treatment. Using the life-cycle model has not helped Chris to think more carefully about the purpose of this project or about who might be the most appropriate sponsor and who the key stakeholders might be.

It appears that the hospital has agreed to put some investment in the project because of Chris being asked to work on the idea, but funding will be required, at least to cover the cost of the time of everyone who needs to be involved in decision making. An early task might be to estimate the probable time involved, the associated costs and the organisations that might be approached to contribute to the budget. In a project that concerns the interests of older patients, how will the service users be represented?

---

The model has helped to identify the amount of work that needs to be put into the early phases in this project. It also demonstrates that planning and implementation will not necessarily follow in a neat sequence. As those involved in the different services meet to discuss how they might improve their work together, planning and implementation will happen alongside the development of shared understanding. The life-cycle model is often criticised as being too simplistic for use in complex settings because it implies a simple linear progression from one phase to the next. Projects often change as they develop and as more is learnt about how they fit into their setting. In health and social care services the context of any project may be rapidly changing. This change will often impact on a project and flexibility is crucial to success.

Each project life cycle will be different. Real life is more chaotic than this model suggests, but it provides a structure that helps to reduce the chaos by putting boundaries around different stages of the project.

## THE CLASSIC SIX-STAGE PROJECT MANAGEMENT MODEL

The classic six-stage project management model (Figure 2.2) helps us to identify key stages of the project and also to consider how these will be integrated during the activities of the project. The project life cycle assumed that the phases identified would be carried out sequentially, but this model is different in that it assumes that some stages are carried out simultaneously. It assumes that communications must take place throughout the project but also proposes that team building, leading and motivation take place from the point at which the project has been defined until it ends.

In the classic six-stage project management model, the *define* stage is similar to that of the project life-cycle model. In this stage the project is fully discussed with all of the stakeholders and the main objectives are identified and agreed. There might be a formal feasibility study and the costs and time-scales are established. This stage is completed when the project brief has been written and agreed.

The second and third stages follow in parallel. The second stage, *plan*, includes the development of the full project plan with the detail of tasks and schedules, resources needed and budgets, a risk analysis and contingency plans. The plan takes some time to prepare and the third stage, *team building, leading and motivation*, begins during the same period. It is usually helpful to involve the people who will be working on the project in the planning, so it is helpful to think of these stages as running in parallel. The members of the team will have different skills and knowledge to contribute, but the one who is managing the project usually acts as the leader and keeps everyone motivated and focused on achieving the objectives. If the team members

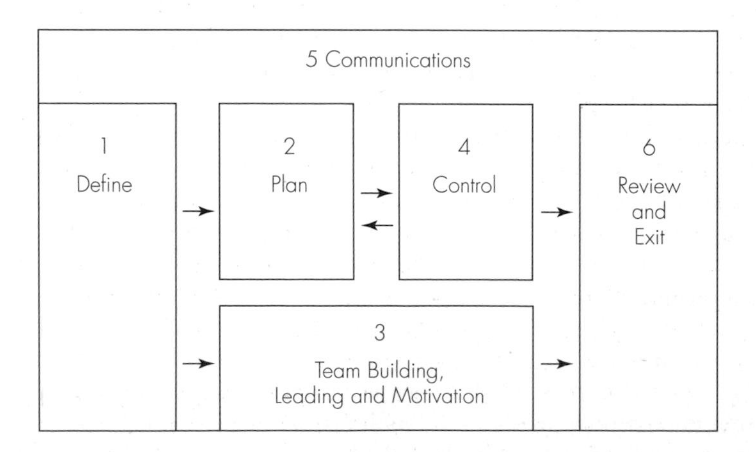


Figure 2.2 The classic six-stage project management model

*Source*: S. Elbeik and M. Thomas, *Project Skills* (Oxford: Butterworth-Heinemann, 1998)

have particular expertise they can often be very helpful in estimating how long the tasks in the plan will take to complete.

The team members are crucial to the next stage, *control*, which can begin once the plan is complete. This stage is the implementation of the project during which all the tasks and activities are carried out and monitored against the plan so that progress can be controlled. Control is essential to ensure that the objectives are completed within the budget and time-scale allowed. Regular reviews are held during this stage to check that everything is progressing according to the plan or to make amendments to the plan if they are needed.

In this model, *communications* take place continuously as a constant feature of the whole process. Communications will be needed both within the project team and between the team and anyone else with a legitimate interest in the project. Some communications will be through formal reporting procedures, but many will be informal.

The final stage is that of *review and exit*. The review is usually concerned to establish that all the objectives were met and to collect information about what can be learnt from the project processes that would be useful to inform future projects.

**Example 2.3 – Using the classic six-stage model**

Once again, Chris made some notes to see whether the classic six-stage model would be helpful in giving those at the scoping meeting an overview of the project and how it might be managed. Here are the notes:

*Define*

I realise now that I need to involve a lot of people in defining this project because we will not be able to make much progress unless we can co-operate. We'll need to discuss who the stakeholders are and negotiate access to talk to those in other services and organisations. The service users are also important stakeholders and we'll need to involve them in discussions, perhaps through representative groups.

Objectives are another problem. I understood originally that the hospital's main interest was in freeing up the beds and helping those who were ready to get back home to their normal lives. We had talked about staffing levels and skills mix in the ward and identifying training and development needs. The only mention of costs was in relation to the costs of using bank and agency staff when we are short of nursing staff. Now I realise that we can't do something like this without working with all the services that provide support and help once people have left hospital.

It might be difficult to set clear objectives with so many potential stake holders, but I suppose we need to do that before we can estimate time and costs for doing what is needed to achieve the objectives. I hadn't thought of doing a feasibility study, but we could discuss that at the meeting. I don't think our hospital thought that the project would involve so many other services and we might need to check that this is the approach that was intended. I think it will take quite a while to get to enough clarity to be able to write a project brief.

*Plan*

We'll not be able to plan in a structured way until we have clear objectives and the time-scale and budget are agreed. I think we might find that working together to clarify the objectives starts us thinking about planning and how we might achieve the outcomes we want. Since planning is ongoing, we'll be able to change our approach if we need to. This means that we probably have to have opportunities to review our progress as we go along, so we might want to decide who should be the core group who make the decisions. It is going to be important to include the team in planning because we don't know enough about each other's areas of work to estimate how long processes take to complete. Even if we decide to develop care plans together, we probably only understand our own area of expertise.

*Team*

I'd thought that we would have a small team with nurses from the ward and perhaps a physiotherapist. I realise now that we'll need to include people from other services, probably a social worker and maybe someone from Primary Care. If we think who has the expertise and skills needed, it has to be a wider team than just the hospital staff.

I've been asked to manage the project, but I think that will also include leadership and motivation as I'll be the only one with substantial time. I hadn't thought about that before, but this will be a new role for me. Perhaps I will be able to find a senior manager in the hospital to mentor me as I'll need some help and support for the role. I don't think that motivation will be too much of an issue if we work together to agree the objectives – it will only get difficult if people think that the hospital is only interested in freeing up the beds.

*Control*

I had been focused on getting started on the implementation but I see now that the objectives must be clear enough for the budget and time-scale to be agreed before even the plan can be made. Once we have a plan, we can still change things, but we'll be able to see how any change impacts on the time-scale and budget. I'll need some sort of steering group to report to if I'm to monitor the progress and make changes, as they might need agreement from higher up if it looks as though the budget or time-scales need to change. I'm only just beginning to understand that the activities will need to be carefully planned so that I can keep some overall control of how the project progresses.

*Communications*

It's clear that we're going to have to set up some good communications arrangements if we are to work across service areas and organisations and keep everyone informed and involved. We'll need ways of informing and consulting all the stakeholders, and there might be different ways for different groups. I'm thinking of the service users again as they won't necessarily be easy to contact on our e-mail. Actually, I don't think the social workers in our area use e-mail either, but maybe some have mobile phones. We'll need to think this through to use appropriate technology and to decide how to inform and how to consult.

*Review and exit*
If we have regular reviews we should be able to hold a final review quite easily. Again, if we have clear objectives we should be able to see whether we have achieved them or not. The exit arrangements should be fairly straightforward if I make a check-list as I think of things that need to be done.

Chris has a better understanding of the scope of the project from using the classic six-stage model. The model has been particularly helpful in showing how the stages needed to be integrated.

---

## ACTIVITY 2.2

What else do you think Chris should do to scope this project?

________________________________________

________________________________________

________________________________________

________________________________________

________________________________________

You might be concerned that there still isn't enough integration. For example, when the team are involved in discussing and agreeing the objectives, they could also be developing the details of the planning and scheduling. They might also have ideas about how the progress could be controlled in a collaborative way once they are able to start implementing the project. There is a danger of letting this project run away if the team start to see what appear to be easy solutions and Chris will need to be quite structured in helping everyone to identify options before rushing into decisions about potential solutions. This model has helped to provide a richer consideration of the stages identified, but in a project that has many strands and multiple outcomes there is still considerable overlap between the stages.

---

Models inevitably offer a simplified view of a situation. They can be helpful in providing a structure to gain an overview of a project, but they do not offer a check-list that will ensure successful completion. They do identify the essential elements, but each project is different. People and teams are always crucial, as they can make the project succeed or fail. Projects usually progress through a series of stages that arise more from the process than either of these models seem to suggest.

Some people think of a project as something that is crafted, like a pot, where planning and doing take place simultaneously and each affects the other.

Projects evolve through a series of loops of planning, acting, reviewing and re-planning. Also, many projects begin without essential information that only becomes available later and often changes the assumptions that have influenced the project until that point. It is important to think of planning as a continuous activity rather than as something that can be completed once and used without change for the duration of the project. Expect change and plan to change the plan.

The first stage of the project is vitally important, as it is the foundation for all the future work. The project needs to be clearly defined so that all of the people involved understand what is to be achieved and why it is worthwhile to carry out the project. It is important to find out who has an interest in the project area and what their interests are. This will help to identify clear objectives and goals for the project. It is also important to establish how much energy and resource should be invested in achieving the results within the time available.

There is no point in going ahead if the project is not likely either to contribute to improvement or to add value in some way, so many projects include an appraisal of the costs and benefits as part of scoping a project. If the project proves to be neither useful nor viable it is better to discover this before much time or resource has been invested, even if you were very committed to the proposal!

CHAPTER 3

# MAKING EVIDENCE-BASED DECISIONS

It is easy to become enthusiastic about a project if it is something that you care about and would like to see achieved. If a project is to attract investment and support, however, it will have to be seen to be both needed and wanted. The key questions are whether the project will achieve what is intended and whether it will work as imagined. There are a number of ways to consider these questions and to assemble the evidence that supports or challenges the ideas that have been proposed.

## DOES THIS PROJECT ADDRESS A NEED?

In health and social care services we are concerned to ensure that we have reliable approaches to identification of needs. These services are focused on addressing immediate needs that are usually made evident through illness or some sort of personal crisis. Identification of needs is important in planning for demand on health and care services and it can reveal focal areas for improvement.

It is not easy to separate needs from wants and demands. When a new miracle drug is publicised, those who believe that it will cure them will want to use it and express a demand for it. However, there will usually be a range of differing opinions about whether it will provide the best cure or whether everyone with the condition would benefit from the treatment. 'Need' is usually applied to something that is fundamental to health and well-being but which may be satisfied in a variety of ways. 'Wants' are more about choices than about meeting a fundamental need. 'Demand' is a forceful expression of a 'want', often including demonstration of need and expression of a choice that is expected to satisfy the need.

In health and social care services resources are limited. In considering whether a project is worth investment, service managers, service users and those responsible for expenditure on service provision will all want to understand how the project will benefit the service user. The benefit may be direct or may be an improvement in an area of service that will ultimately provide a better service or better use of resources. Therefore it is important to consider how the proposed project will make a worthwhile contribution.

### Anticipating needs

The world around us is constantly changing and new needs emerge from changes in our environment. Some of the new needs may be within our own service areas but others will be in the communities we serve. Where there is a need, there will be people with interests of various kinds who will want some action to be taken. It is helpful if those working in health and care services can anticipate and predict emergent needs so that we understand them well enough to respond proactively.

### Recognising needs

A need is recognised when there is evidence that there is a problem that should be addressed. It is usually necessary to collect and present information to demonstrate a need. This might include making use of existing data from both inside and outside service areas, but it usually also involves collection and analysis of additional data. As the need becomes clearly identified there is often some indication of measures that might be taken to address the need. This stage of needs identification is also concerned with beginning to identify the outcomes and outputs that might become the goals of projects that are set up to address the newly identified need.

### Describing needs

Needs can be recognised and described at a number of levels. Health and care needs are identified for whole regions in funding plans but teams of staff in health and social care are often involved in identifying and planning to meet needs in their own areas of work.

Before anything can be done to address the need, it has to be described in a way that enables everyone to understand the problem. This includes describing its characteristics and explaining why it is important to take action. It may be helpful to work with groups and individuals who have an interest in the new area of need to ensure that it has been thoroughly understood. This activity should lead to a precise statement of the need and, eventually, to a proposal of what must be done or provided to meet the need. If the action to be taken is a project, this statement will contribute to the formal definition of the project.

## DOES IT HELP US TO ACHIEVE OUR ORGANISATIONAL GOALS?

If a project is successful it will achieve its own objectives and also fit in with the strategic plans of the organisation. A project will usually attract support if it will help others to achieve their objectives and if it will help to move the work of the organisation in the right direction.

In the very early stages of a project there is an opportunity to consider whether it is as well aligned as it could be with the objectives of the organisation or service area. It is not unusual to focus a proposal on showing how the project can achieve the outcomes intended, but to forget to ensure that the project and its outcomes fit well with other developments that are taking place. Discuss with the project sponsor how much the project will contribute to progressing organisational objectives. It is often possible to address a slightly wider range of concerns if this is planned as part of defining the project – but it is difficult to do it later in the planning stage.

The questions that will help you to determine the value of the project to the organisation are:

- How will this project help us to carry out our purpose more effectively?
- How exactly will the project contribute to achieving any of the organisation's stated objectives?

In health and care organisations it is also advisable to ask:

- How will this project contribute to improving the service for the patient or user?

If you ask these questions of the project and find that it does not contribute directly, the feasibility of the project should be considered as doubtful because the use of resources will be difficult to justify.

**Example 3.1 – Aligning with the business plan**

In the early 1990s two NHS Management Training and Development Departments based in the West Midlands were merged. For two years the newly formed department provided an unchanged menu of fairly standard short courses. However, the changing climate of the NHS in the mid 1990s placed pressure on the department to deliver new forms of learning and development.

The Head of Training and Development along with the Director of Human Resources had several meetings to discuss the situation. The Head of Training and Development knew that the organisational business plan had several objectives. These hinged on her department delivering certain outcomes including appraisal training, recruitment and selection training, change management and business planning skills. A more significant change was the expectation that staff would change their roles from 'trainers' to internal consultants and facilitators to help individual managers solve problems, manage change and build effective teams.

The Head involved her own staff from an early stage and also decided that they would be key decision makers in how the department could adapt to meet changing and challenging objectives. She informed her staff about her meeting with the Director of HR and the content of her discussions. She did not present a *fait accompli* but an opportunity for her staff to explore. Several were immediately excited by the prospect of change and the opportunity for personal growth, while others took a more cautious view.

Then the Head met individually with members of staff to ascertain their views and to answer any questions they might have. The meetings generally progressed very well. The issues raised mainly concerned lack of skills and knowledge in the new areas of work. One idea that came from the staff was to have an 'away day'. The purpose of the away day was to share ideas, assess the team's strengths and develop a vision for the future. The objectives of the day were met and the team started to develop a plan for implementing the shared vision. The team met at their regular staff meeting two days later and agreed to focus on a single agenda item of developing the project plan.

The Head went with two of her staff to present the plan to the Director of HR, who was very impressed with the attitude of the staff and the ideas that they had agreed. An estimate had been made of the resourcing necessary to implement the plan, with costs of retraining, skills acquisition and visits to other departments in the region. The Director of HR invited the Head and her staff to present their ideas at the next Trust Board meeting. Although slightly daunted, the staff agreed. Two weeks later the plan was formally presented to the Board of Directors, who fully supported the ideas presented and agreed to fund and fully resource the plan.

(Stephen Oliver, Management Training Consultant,
Business Development Consultancy)

## HAVE WE CONSIDERED ALL OF THE OPTIONS?

As we ask whether the project will work or not, we often find that previously unconsidered options emerge. We might realise that there are other ways of achieving the same outcome or we might have become aware of new perspectives that raise questions about aspects of the project and cause us to consider different options.

One way of generating options is to seek other ideas, perhaps from your colleagues or from the stakeholders in the issues addressed by the project. One way to collect ideas is to have a 'brainstorming' session. This is usually done with small groups in which one person writes up the ideas on a flip chart. Everyone is encouraged to call out any ideas they have and it is important to stress that others should not judge or comment on the ideas at that stage, because if people are allowed to offer criticism it can stop individuals from offering creative or unusual ideas. At the end of a brainstorming session you might discuss the ideas and even build on some of them or dismiss some completely.

However you do it, it is usual to consider what options exist before the final decision is taken about investing in a project. There is always the option to do nothing and it is worth considering what the outcome would be if nothing at all was done to intervene.

If there appear to be a number of possible options and a decision has to be made about which direction to choose, it can be helpful to carry out an option appraisal.

## Option appraisal

The purpose of an option appraisal is to decide which is the best option to choose to achieve your purpose. You can't carry out an option appraisal until you have a very clear description of the purpose. Ideally, this description will include objectives and criteria by which success can be judged.

Draw up a set of criteria by which you can judge whether each option would achieve your objectives. The criteria usually include any limits that have to be placed on costs, time, who carries out the work, where the work is carried out and how the quality of outcome will be ensured. If the decision is difficult to make once these criteria have been considered, you can take each of the criteria and rank them in order according to importance. The best option will be the one that meets the highest number of the most important criteria. Another way to judge it is to give each option a score for each of the criteria it meets, perhaps marking one out of ten if many of the criteria are not fully met. Then you can identify the best option by adding the scores achieved by each one.

Using numerical scales to help in making these judgements may seem strange as there is no basis other than judgement for awarding the scores. The advantage of using these methods is that it forces you to consider the strengths of each option from a number of different perspectives. We often have a preference and are not always sure why we prefer one option to another, so it can be important to test our initial judgements by using a method that might challenge our impressions. At times we may find that a favourite option does not perform well when tested against other options. This is sometimes because we have not included all the criteria that we want to use in making the judgement. For example, in some settings it is very important that people who share the values of those in the setting carry out a project. If this is important, it should be added to the list of criteria. We often make judgements using a range of not only openly expressed criteria but also a few criteria that have not been fully understood or discussed. Many would argue that the best decisions are made when the criteria have been very carefully prepared so that the process can be seen to be 'transparent'.

## COST-EFFECTIVENESS

A cost-effectiveness analysis enables you to compare the different costs involved in each optional way of achieving the same objectives or outcome. The option that costs the least would normally be considered to be the most cost-effective. This method is only useful if the outcome has been described thoroughly. For example, if a project is intended to achieve some staff development during the process it would not be more cost-effective to hire temporary staff. This option would not have been considered if staff development had been identified as an objective of the project. It is very important to be explicit about all of the objectives and goals of the project before applying any financial tests. Sometimes projects are so strongly supported by people convinced of their worth that it becomes very difficult to make an unbiased appraisal of whether the organisation would or would not benefit. Sometimes there are conflicting values and loyalties that exaggerate the anticipated benefits. Once the objectives and goals are clear the application of financial tests can help to ensure that decisions taken about investment in the project will stand up to scrutiny by those whose money is being invested.

## OPPORTUNITIES AND THREATS

Some people will see the project as offering opportunities and others will see threats. Those who see opportunities may sometimes want to include additional aims and objectives and it is important to consider where the boundaries of the project are. The answer often lies in having a clear statement of the purpose of the project. This will enable you to identify what has to be done to achieve that purpose. For example, service improvements often raise the question of whether additional training should be provided. If the purpose of the project is clear, it will be possible to identify what has to be provided in order to enable staff to do what is necessary to achieve the purpose. However, the opportunity to provide additional training might be worth considering if that would make good use of resources or help to achieve the wider goals of the organisation. It is important to discuss the opportunities before the project brief is written so that they can be incorporated if they add value without diverting the project from its core purpose.

The disruption that a project might bring is often seen as a threat. These fears include disruption to services or to the working lives of individuals. If full discussions are held with the people who might be affected by the project, they can be encouraged to express their fears. There will not always be easy solutions that will be seen to reduce the fear, but if the feelings are respected and discussed there is an opportunity to judge the extent to which the fears present a threat to the project. Some fears may reveal threats that had not been previously considered and may be vital in helping to shape the project in a way that can be successful. Other fears may prove to be unjustified and can be reviewed as the project progresses.

## IS THIS PROJECT FEASIBLE?

If a project is large or innovative, you might carry out a feasibility study before beginning the detailed work of planning and implementation. A feasibility study considers whether the project can achieve what is intended within the setting and resources available. If there are different ways in which the project might be carried out, a feasibility study can help to clarify which option or options would achieve the objectives in the most beneficial way.

The key issues to consider in a feasibility study are:

- *Values.* In health and care services it is very important to check that the intended processes and outcomes of the project align with the values of the service area and the setting of that service. In particular, will this project deliver a benefit for service users? For example, it would not be appropriate to carry out a project in a way that would disadvantage some service users in a setting in which there was an overall intention to promote equality or to improve health.
- *Finance.* Compare the cost of all the resources that will be necessary to carry out the project with the benefits the project is intended to bring. The basic question is whether the project is worth doing. Also consider the cost of not doing the project, as there may be penalties if your service area does not develop as quickly as new policies or other conditions require it to.
- *Technical.* This includes not only the technical aspects of completing the project but also the 'fit' of the project with its surroundings. Consider the way any new system or technology will fit with existing systems and whether staff have the competence to use the new system. There may be a need to plan for training and a transition period. Also consider whether the proposed new system or technology is the best for the purpose intended and whether enough work has been done to identify alternatives.
- *Ecological.* Consider the potential impact of the project, both as it is carried out and its outcomes, on the local environment and local social conditions. The project has not only to fit well within the organisation or service area, but also to be acceptable to those in your immediate locality. The environmental impact is also very important and worth considering at an early stage so that you can plan to be as responsive as possible to concerns that might be raised. Areas to consider are whether your project might cause more traffic or noise, lead to an increased need for parking, threaten wildlife or open 'green' areas or impact in any way on local concerns.
- *Social.* Another consideration is whether the project will attract support from staff and service users and from the general public.

Will the project improve or impact on social settings or relationships? Both the processes used and the intended outcomes can be reviewed in terms of whether there is an opportunity to make the project more attractive and useful so that it is well supported. For example, it might be possible to offer some training to those who carry out the project or to involve local people in helping to shape services in ways that would be beneficial to the community.

- *People management*. Consider whether there will be any implications for work practices and how you might plan for appropriate consultation with staff, particularly if there might be any changes to terms and conditions of employment. There is often a training and development aspect if the project is intended to contribute to organisational change. Consider how equal opportunities will be addressed and whether any special measures should be taken before, during or after the project.

It may not take very long to carry out a feasibility study for a project that has limited call on resources and a clearly defined outcome that is agreed to be necessary. It is often possible to do this in informal discussions if a project is small and uncontroversial. For a larger project, however, it is usual to have a very comprehensive feasibility study to avoid investment in something that may not be worthwhile.

**Example 3.2 – A feasibility study**

Managers in a Primary Care Clinic decided that its patients and the local general public would benefit from a directory of all services with information about how to contact each service. The group conducted a feasibility study. The areas considered were:

- How the directory could be genuinely accessible to all service users in terms of language, format, accessibility and understandability. This was important in order to address equality of opportunity. They also considered whether they would be meeting the full purpose of their organisation if they failed to offer a comprehensive directory.
- The cost of collecting and presenting the information and the ongoing costs involved in keeping the directory up to date. Options of using leaflets, noticeboards, telephone helplines, prerecorded telephone messages and web pages were considered. The benefits of using different methods and the potential to use a range of languages were considered. The cost of not providing the information was also considered.
- There were a number of technical considerations. The clinic already had an information system that could be accessed by staff but not by service users. There were already reception services and a telephone help-

line, but the staff that worked in these areas had complained that they often had to give out information that could be readily available in other forms.

- There was some concern about part of the proposal that involved providing a help desk separate from the reception area in the clinic. There was already little space for the waiting area and queues often formed at the reception desk. There was also a fear that the limited parking space outside the clinic would be taken up by people calling in for information rather than those with appointments.
- They considered whether similar projects had been successful elsewhere in terms of benefits to the local community without putting too much strain on the normal workings of a clinic.
- There was consideration of whether the proposed project manager had the time and expertise to manage the project. The more it was discussed, the more complex it seemed to become. It was also recognised that support would be required from the clinic staff and from other agencies in the area for data collection.

## SHOULD WE DO A PILOT STUDY?

If the proposed project is on a large scale, or if considerable expense is anticipated, it is often a good idea to try the ideas out in a pilot study. If you are planning a pilot study it is important to remember that the main purpose of this is to learn as much as possible to inform the proposed substantial project. This means that a pilot study needs to be planned to enable appropriate learning. There is no point in carrying out a pilot study if the process cannot inform future projects, for example, if each setting in which the project will be run is so different that the project must be planned differently for each.

There are two ways in which pilot studies are frequently designed:

1 The pilot attempts to carry out the whole range of project activities leading to the full range of outcomes, but does this in only one situation or geographical area. This sort of pilot is often used to try out a large-scale project that can be piloted and revised before running it on the large scale. For example, a project to introduce a new induction process might be piloted in one department or area of work before being implemented across a whole organisation.
2 The pilot tests only a part of the final project. For example, if the project includes use of new technology, the project team might attempt a small task to learn more about the technology before starting a project that relies on its use.

**Example 3.3 – Setting up a pilot study**

A Directorate Manager was responsible for a project that included devolving budget responsibility to unit levels. This meant that budgets would have to be managed at levels further down the organisation than had been the practice previously. Although she had personal experience of managing at the unit level, this was at a time when budgets had not been devolved and she was worried about whether she could anticipate all the issues that might arise. She decided to run a pilot study with a small group of the unit managers who were most interested and most motivated, so that they could be involved in developing systems that would work effectively. She also hoped that this approach would help her to learn more about how 'housekeeping' could be improved at unit level.

It is often a good idea to involve people who are interested in pilot studies because it helps to establish what is possible without having to work with people who are reluctant and who might create unnecessary obstacles.

As a pilot study is designed as a learning process it is important to set objectives that indicate what you are trying to learn. Attempting to write such objectives will often help to determine whether it is likely to be helpful to run a pilot or whether it might be better simply to start the project but to build in frequent review events to ensure that you learn from your work as you progress.

## IS THE BENEFIT WORTH THE COST?

Any project involves the transformation of *inputs* into an *output*. The work of the project team, the materials and other resources that they use and the energy that they put into the project all contribute to the transformation that is the overall *outcome* of the project, the change that the project has produced. For example, the inputs to a project might include a small team of people who gather information and make a display (using a wide range of materials) for an exhibition to publicise the services they offer. The outputs of the project would include the exhibition materials that had been created and, maybe, a list of contacts that had been made during the exhibition. Overall outcomes of the project would be wider and include any new service users whose awareness of the service has been raised by the exhibition and the team's capability of being able to take part in a similar exhibition again.

One aspect of carrying out a cost–benefit analysis is to ask questions about the relationship of inputs to outputs and outcomes. The most basic questions to ask are:

- What resources will be required and how much will these cost?
- What outputs or outcomes will be produced?
- What will be the quality of outcomes and outputs?
- What quantities will be produced?

The aim of asking these questions is to identify the cost of the project, the cost of transforming inputs into outputs and outcomes. It is important to try to express the proposed outcomes clearly because projects in health and social care are not always intended to produce things that can be counted and then costed as separate items. You might be planning service improvements or changes that will make processes or procedures more effective. Whatever the project is, there will be costs if the thinking and work are carried out in time that could be used for something else.

In large-scale projects there are several financial measures that would usually be used to test the financial viability of the proposal. There will be consideration of how the cash flow during the project will impact on the organisation and whether any financial value will be gained. The aim of using financial tests is to ensure that those who take decisions about whether to undertake the project or not are fully informed of the financial implications. The consideration of whether investment in the project is likely to be worthwhile has to be considered in relation to the short-term and long-term financial prospects of the organisation. The demands of a project on the cash flow of an organisation can have an impact on other areas of work unless the demands have been anticipated and provision made to cover the additional finance required. If money has to be borrowed, this may incur additional costs and the period required to repay the loan will also have to be considered.

Sometimes the costs are 'hidden' because the project can be carried out as part of existing work. We might propose that a project that does not require additional staff does not have a staff cost. However, this is a false argument because staff are employed with job descriptions and agreed areas of work. If you ask them to do something different instead of what they would normally be doing, this represents a cost to the organisation because you are, in effect, employing the staff to carry out different work. In some circumstances this might be acceptable, for example if the flow of work leaves gaps during which it is difficult to keep staff fully occupied (which is rather unlikely in very busy health and care services!). In other circumstances it might indicate that workloads are not very carefully monitored and there is a danger of overloading some individuals.

Once the cost of the project has been estimated, it is possible to consider the value of the project. If something that you intend to sell has been produced, you have to decide on a price for the product. The price is not necessarily very closely related to the cost because pricing is related to what the intended purchaser will pay. For example, you might have produced a very effective reading aid for children that many people want and would buy at a low price but not at a high price. If you find that you can only produce it at a high cost you will still not be able to sell the product at a high price. However, if you can produce these items at a low cost and sell them at a slightly higher but still low enough price you have the possibility of generating revenue. This project might still not work if the quantities that can be produced do not match the quantities that can be sold. There might also be costs that had not been considered related to the storage of products and the sales processes, including packaging and delivery. These issues must be considered even in non-profit organisations if the intention is simply to cover costs by selling at cost price. The cost often includes more than we expect, particularly if we are expecting to carry out the project within the 'slack' of the organisation's resources.

The value of the project might be difficult to express in monetary terms if it is more about improving something that is already available, for example a service improvement. In some cases it is easy to identify a potential saving in time or resources and these can be costed. However, if your proposed project is intended to improve the quality of experience, this is much more difficult to express as a value. You might be able to express the value in terms of the benefit to the service user, particularly if it would potentially reduce their reliance on services in future by increasing their ability to be more independent. There might be a wider benefit in terms of the effects of better experience on other service users. For example, if a parent has a traumatic experience at the dentist, it is difficult for them to encourage their children to go to the dentist. This also raises the possibility that the value of the project might be related to the potential cost of not doing it. If this is the case, you can use that potential cost to explain the expected value of carrying out the project.

Project costs are usually divided into development costs and operational costs. The development costs arise during the project and include the staff and other resources required to produce the project outputs. Once there are some outputs, there may be operational costs. These are costs associated with maintaining or using the project outputs. For example, if the project has involved setting up a new computerised system, there will be ongoing maintenance costs and there might also be staff training costs that would not have arisen without the change caused by the project.

In projects that are tested by a formal feasibility study there will be formal costings of all aspects of the project. The aim is to ensure that the project outcome contributes greater value than the value of the resources that would be used in completing the project. This economic measure is not the only one that would be considered as the context is very important. If the project would contribute to achieving the purpose of the organisation, this would offer a powerful argument in its favour. For many health and care organisations, another powerful argument would arise if a project was wanted and supported by the local community or general public.

We have considered a number of ways in which you might gather evidence to support (or not support) project proposals. If you find that the evidence does support the project ideas, this work will provide a sound foundation for development of the project brief.

CHAPTER 4

# DEFINING THE PROJECT

Once the scope of the project has become clear and there is a commitment to go ahead, it is neccessary to define the project as a written document. This might be called 'terms of reference', 'project definition document' or 'project brief'. The purpose of the project brief (or similar document) is to detail exactly what the project is intended to produce and the resources and constraints within which it must be achieved. This document is almost always signed by the sponsor of the project – the person who is funding the project or who holds responsibility for the use of resources to achieve the outcomes identified. The process of drawing up the brief can help to clarify areas that had not previously been fully discussed and often demonstrates that there is more work to do before the brief can be completed.

## WORKING WITH THE SPONSOR

The sponsor is the person or group who has commissioned the project and put you in charge of managing it. In most workplace projects there are costs of staff time and resources that must be funded. The sponsor is the person who has ultimate responsibility for the funding and who will say whether the project has or has not been successful in meeting its goals.

As the sponsor has such an important role, it is worth ensuring that you have completely understood what the sponsor is expecting the project to achieve. This is not always easy. It is worth checking out your understanding in several different ways so that you are fully informed before you set off into detailed planning. If you are planning to achieve the objectives that you think are appropriate and you discover at a later date that your project sponsor had different ideas and was imagining different outcomes, it will usually be very difficult to bring the differences to a satisfactory resolution.

Even when you have agreed the broad goals and the detailed objectives of a project with your sponsor, you might find that events at a later date cause you to revisit this agreement. This is why it is so important to have a written agreement as a basis for the project planning. The agreement, the project brief, is your licence to act on behalf of the sponsor. If you deviate from that agreement without consulting the sponsor and seeking an amendment to the agreement, you are in breach of the contract. This may sound very formal, but the project brief details the contract made between you and the sponsor. The sponsor has to be accountable for his or her use of the organisation's resources and has, in essence, delegated some of that responsibility to you. The project brief details the extent of this delegated responsibility and you are accountable to the sponsor for the use of resources to achieve the goals agreed.

It is very unlikely that you will be able to complete the project without making any changes to the project brief because it is impossible to foresee everything that may impinge on the project as it is implemented. The important thing is to keep working with the sponsor as you become aware of any potential changes so that you can decide together how to respond and whether to change the project brief. If you do decide to change the brief, it is important to document the nature of the change and to obtain the sponsor's signature to demonstrate that the change has been agreed and authorised. As before, this is so that if there is any dispute about whether the project has achieved its aims there will be a document that details exactly what was agreed, against which the outcomes can be assessed.

You will probably have realised that it is helpful to keep in regular contact with your sponsor so that there are no surprises as the project develops. In some cases, the sponsor may prefer you to work closely with someone he or she appoints to monitor the project and you should then treat them as you would the sponsor.

If you are carrying out a project that is essentially your own idea and something that you want to do and have the means to carry out without drawing on additional resources, you may feel that your project does not have a sponsor. It is worth considering whether you could ask someone to act in that capacity anyway, so that you have a 'sounding board' to discuss the project with. Even if all the aspects of the project fall within your own areas of responsibility, you are still committing the organisation's resources if you are spending your own work time on the project. If you can gain the support of a more senior manager to act as the project sponsor it will ensure that you have the approval of your organisation to carry out the project. It might also be more beneficial to the organisation if your project helps others to consider alternative ways of achieving objectives and you might find that your idea becomes a pilot project for eventual wider use.

## WILL THE PROJECT BE SUPPORTED?

It is important to consider a wide range of views before starting any detailed planning, whether the project is small or large. It is helpful to consult all the people who might be affected by the project, all of the people who hold a stake in the process or outcomes – the stakeholders. Stakeholders will include the sponsor or client of the project, anyone whose resources will be needed to carry out the project, anyone who will contribute their work, time or energy to the project and anyone who will be affected by the process or outcomes. This is often a large number of people and you might want to consider how to hear representative views from groups of stakeholders.

**Example 4.1 – Issues identified in developing a project brief**

A large Acute Hospitals NHS Trust in the Midlands had recently merged with a smaller Acute Trust and as part of the restructuring fifteen Clinical Director posts were created. After several months the organisation's perception was that these new Clinical Directors were struggling to implement the managerial element of their role. The solution seemed simple, which was to design a management development programme specifically aimed at improving and developing the managerial knowledge and skills of these Clinical Directors. However, before this action was taken the Organisational Development Manager decided to interview a random sample of Clinical Directors to help identify precise needs. During these interviews it became apparent that a number of Clinical Directors felt a need for development around the following areas:

- conflict management
- performance management
- budgetary management
- time management.

To some extent these areas could have been anticipated, but a number of other issues were also identified. These included:

- role clarification
- understanding of the new organisation
- relationship building and networking
- an understanding of the wider world, the government's agenda and how to respond effectively to targets and demands.

Some of these needs had come as a surprise, yet clearly these issues, which may have seemed basic such as 'what exactly does my role as Clinical Director entail?' were of real concern to the individuals involved. This enabled a programme of development to be designed which was targeted at improving the skills and knowledge areas identified by the Clinical Directors, rather than basing this on assumptions and providing something less relevant.

(Stephen Oliver, Management Training Consultant, Business Development Consultancy)

People are sometimes reluctant to seek opinions from stakeholders who might disapprove of the project. We might sometimes think that it is better not to encourage discussion of controversial issues until the project is more advanced. We sometimes don't even realise that there will be opposition to an idea that seems a good one from our own perspective. It is worth considering the consequences of not understanding the opposition to a project. Much of the concern about a project can be anticipated and avoided if the views of stakeholders are understood at an early stage.

## STAKEHOLDER MAPPING

You need to identify who your stakeholders are before you can consider the impact that they might have on the project. Stakeholders will include:

- The *sponsor* or *client* – the person or people who have commissioned or authorised the project and who will provide resources. This person will also usually be the one who confirms that the project has been successfully completed.
- The *project team* – the people who will carry out all of the tasks and activities to complete the project. These people will need to have the knowledge, skills and experience to achieve the goals of the project. They also need to be available to work on the project at the right time.
- Other *managers in the organisation* – particularly line managers of people who have been seconded to the project team and functional managers who control resources that will be needed. You will often have to negotiate with these people to ensure that your project team and other resources are available at the right time.
- *Individuals and groups who will be affected* by the project. These will include people who are interested in either the process of the project (for example people whose lives may be disrupted as project tasks are carried out) and people who may gain advantages or be disadvantaged by the outcomes of the project. Service users and patients might be considered as a stakeholder group.
- *Individuals and groups who hold direct influence* over the project. It is important to identify anyone or any group who hold the power to damage or stop the project. These are powerful stakeholders whose particular concerns may lead them to use their power to help or hinder the project. Ask the question, 'Who could stop this project?' For example, who could withhold funding or prevent access to labour or resources?
- People who act as *representatives of the general public* or of groups with interests in the project. These may include elected representatives in local government, trustees in a charitable trust or non-executive directors, local residents' groups (especially if the project involves a new service provision or changes to locations of services). The media will give attention to projects that will interest the general public and

you may need to provide information to local newspapers, radio and television.

- Other *organisations*. If your project involves changes to service provision, other organisations may be stakeholders. For example, voluntary organisations may provide services linking or complementary to those of your organisation. There may also be organisations who provide similar services and compete for resources or service users or who collaborate with your organisation to provide opportunities for choice in your locality.
- *Professional bodies*, *institutes*, *trade unions* or *any other formal organisation* that may have interests because of the nature of the project. If the project involves developments that link in any way with agreed procedures or policies these bodies may want to be consulted.

Each of these stakeholders or groups will have different expectations of the project and will offer support or opposition according to how they perceive the project. There may be conflict in these different views and not all stakeholders will be open in expressing their views, especially if they are not asked to comment. The first you might hear of a problem could be when someone complains in a very public forum. You do not, however, need to wait anxiously for this to happen – you can manage the project in a way that anticipates a difference in views and provides opportunities for these to be expressed at an early stage and ideally before the project brief is completed.

Many formal project management methodologies, such as PRINCE, have formalised procedures for dealing with sponsor and stakeholder issues through a project board structure and regular meetings. PRINCE (PRojects IN Controlled Environments) is a structured method for effective project management. It is used extensively by UK government organisations and is widely recognised and used in the private sector, both in the UK and internationally. The key features of PRINCE are:

- its focus on business justification;
- its defined organisation structure set out for the project management team;
- its product-based planning approach that emphasises outcomes;
- its emphasis on dividing the project into manageable and controllable stages;
- its flexibility to be applied at a level appropriate to the project.

Whether or not you use a formal methodology such as PRINCE, it is useful to identify the stakeholders of the project and to review the extent of influence that they might have on the project. It is often helpful to work with other people to identify the stakeholders to ensure that a wide range of different viewpoints are included in your final list.

**Example 4.2 – Stakeholders in a new record-keeping system**

A project that involves developing and implementing a new record-keeping system in a community health or social care service will involve people who provide and record data, people who store and retrieve the data and people who use the data. The stakeholders for the project will include:

- receptionists, clerks and others who collect and record the data;
- patients and service users who provide the data (and any special interest groups who are concerned about how data are collected for any reason);
- those who file and retrieve the data when they are required;
- those who ensure that records are kept confidential;
- those who use the records to make service provision decisions (for example professionals, nurses, health workers, doctors and others);
- those who use the records to make financial decisions;
- those who use the records to review service provision levels;
- those who use the records to plan for use of equipment and materials;
- those who ensure that the system works (whether electronic or paper-based);
- anyone who will have to transfer records from the old system to the new one (this might be a very significant role if there are large numbers of records to transfer);
- managers who have to reschedule staff responsibilities to enable the project to take place;
- any new staff who are recruited to the project team;
- other organisations and staff in those organisations who regularly require data from your organisation or who provide data to your organisation.

Some people who like the existing system may not want any change and so will oppose or be difficult because they see the project as causing unnecessary work. Some individuals and groups may see the opportunity to collect data in a way that is more convenient for service users or in more appropriate ways for people with particular concerns or needs. Record-keeping systems are used in so many different ways by so many different interests that a project that involves any change to the system may upset a surprising number of people.

Each setting and project proposal will have different stakeholders and different concerns. You may find it useful to make a 'stakeholder map' to work out the stakeholders for your project. An example is given in Figure 4.1. This stakeholder map is for a project that involves making physical and process changes to a reception and waiting area in a hospital. The changes will affect the provision of several services in the hospital and also the transport and parking arrangements.

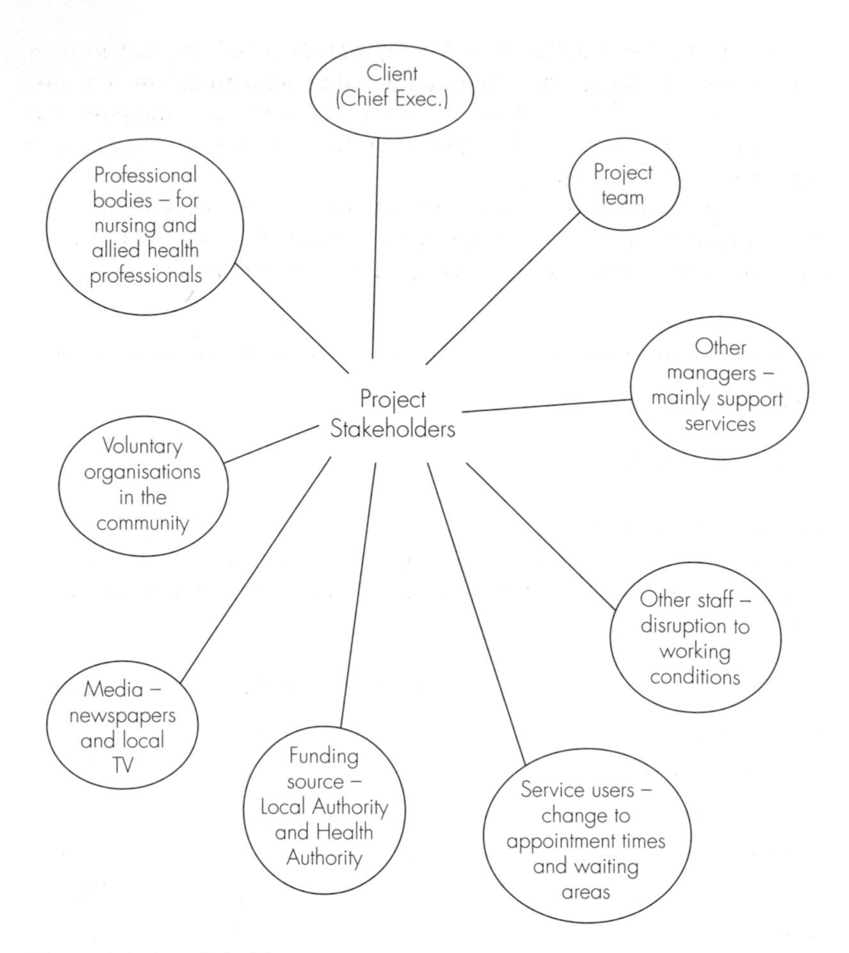


Figure 4.1 A stakeholder map

# WORKING WITH YOUR STAKEHOLDERS

Those managing a project are usually interested in trying to gain as much support as possible for the project so that the stakeholders assist the progress of the project or, at least, so that they don't delay or interrupt the schedule. Ideally, you will also want the stakeholders to lend their verbal support during the project and to express satisfaction with the outcomes. As all the stakeholders will have their own hopes and fears relating to the project, it is not easy to gain complete support. There is an opportunity to listen to these hopes and fears at a very early stage when the project is first proposed. It is easier to ask for reactions at this stage than at a later stage when commitments have been made. You will be aware of the obstacles that may face the project and be well informed about the different views of each stakeholder or group and their different priorities. Once you have heard their hopes and fears you may be able to plan to include outcomes that will satisfy more of the hopes than were included in the original ideas and you may also be able to reduce the impact of the outcomes that are feared. You may not be able to meet all of the expectations or to avoid all of the potential problems, but you will be in a good position to plan how to manage perceptions of the project.

One way of thinking about how different stakeholders might react is to consider whether there are differences in how they might view each of the key dimensions of budget, schedule and quality.

## ACTIVITY 4.1

*Allow 5 minutes.*

Consider the different views each of these stakeholders might have of the three key dimensions of a project. Put a tick to indicate which dimension each stakeholder might think is the most important from their personal perspective.

| | *Budget* | *Schedule* | *Quality* |
|---|---|---|---|
| Project sponsor | ❒ | ❒ | ❒ |
| Functional expert | ❒ | ❒ | ❒ |
| Line manager | ❒ | ❒ | ❒ |
| Supplier or contractor | ❒ | ❒ | ❒ |
| Patient or service user | ❒ | ❒ | ❒ |
| Project team | ❒ | ❒ | ❒ |
| Project manager | ❒ | ❒ | ❒ |

The *sponsor* usually focuses on the budget and the outcomes. What return is achieved for the investment? What financial risks are involved and is it achieving value for money? As the outcomes are produced, the focus of a sponsor may change to concern about the quality, about ensuring that the outcomes are well received by patients or service users. The sponsor is less likely to be interested in the schedule as long as the overall time-scales that were agreed are met.

A *functional expert* (for example an accountant or surveyor or trainer) is likely to be focused on the quality of work, both the work associated with the project and the impact of the project requirements on any other work in progress. Thus the functional expert will be concerned to balance the quality of outcomes with the schedule and will want to have sufficient time to achieve high-quality results.

A *line manager* is likely not to be directly involved in the project, but to be responsible for staff who are members of the project team. This manager's interest will probably be to ensure that the project schedule will not be too disruptive of other work. The staffing resource will usually need to be agreed with any line managers of people that you would like to include in the project team.

*Suppliers and contractors* are required to fit in with the schedule to provide whatever is contracted at the right time and place. Their concern is usually to ensure that the budget has allowed them to make a profit or to achieve their service goals and that they are able to provide the required quality of goods or services within the schedule allowed. Thus suppliers and contractors have to balance these three dimensions but also to ensure that the agreement represents value for their business or area of work.

*Patients and service users* often want the outcome quickly and may apply pressure to speed up the schedule, but once the outcomes are delivered the focus from this perspective moves to the quality. If the project has been scheduled tightly to meet the expectations of service users it will still be essential to meet the quality requirements if the project is to be considered a success.

The staff who form the *project team* will have concerns about all of the project dimensions, depending on the nature of each person's contribution. If they can be encouraged to work as a team and to understand the tensions caused by the time-scale, budget and quality requirements they may help the project manager to keep the dimensions balanced.

The *project manager* has to balance all three dimensions and to accommodate the different priorities put on each by different stakeholders at different times.

---

The project manager can demonstrate the interdependency of the dimensions, both to help the team members to understand and collaborate and also to show stakeholders that putting an emphasis on any one dimension will have consequences for the others. For example, if the schedule is to be reduced or the quality is to be enhanced, a case could be made for the budget to be increased. However, in very large projects many different teams may be contributing to the project and it may not be possible for them to work closely together. There may not be a team at all in the sense of planning and working closely together – some projects are accomplished by groups of specialists co-ordinated by those managing the project.

## CREATING THE PROJECT BRIEF

Whether you define your project in a document called 'terms of reference' or a 'project definition document', it usually incorporates a section consisting of a detailed project brief. The project brief is the essential record of what has been agreed with those responsible for funding the project and it will be the document that you have to return to if there is any dispute about what has been achieved once the project is in its final stages. It is very important to construct the project brief carefully because it is the basis for all further work on the project. It is the document that underpins all later decision making and planning.

The project brief is essentially a record of an agreement about the main concerns of the project. It is usually the responsibility of the person managing the project to draft it after consulting the sponsor and key stakeholders. It reflects the three dimensions of a project in its key areas:

- the outcomes expected of the project (the quality dimension);
- the resources that will be invested to achieve the outcomes (the budget dimension);
- the time that will be taken to complete the project (the time dimension).

Although it may take a long time and a lot of discussion before the project brief can be drafted, the document itself should be concise and clear. It should detail exactly what should be achieved by the project and give practical details about how this will be achieved. It is important that the document be clear and unambiguous because much of the planning will be based on this brief. It is also the document that will be used to revise the agreement if any changes are necessary as the project progresses. It is also usual to include guidelines about how decisions will be made, identifying levels of authority and procedures to be followed.

## STRUCTURE OF THE PROJECT BRIEF

As the project brief should be clear and concise, it usually has headings and lists. It is a summary record of the agreements on which the project is based. A check-list of the headings that you will need is given in Figure 4.2.

In a complex project there might be previous documents outlining initial decisions. These can be referred to rather than repeated in the project brief and may be added as appendices. There may be documents about the background to the project and the justification for expenditure. Key objectives need to be put into the project brief, but detailed objectives are usually identified later when the project plan is developed. The criteria for success are important as they help to check that you all have a similar picture of what success will mean. These are also the measures that will be used to check whether the project achieved its objectives.

The project brief will indicate some of the scheduling concerns in the project. The date for completion will have been identified along with the key deliverables and when they will be handed over. Most projects also agree a schedule for reviewing progress, either monthly or quarterly, depending on the length of the project. The things that should have been achieved at each of these review stages are usually called

Project title
Name of sponsor or other contact responsible for project approval
Locations – addresses of sponsor, project location, contact addresses
Name of person managing the project and contact details
Date of agreement of project brief
Date of project start and finish
Background to the project and purpose with goals outlined
Key objectives with quality and success criteria
Details of how achievement of these will bring benefits to the sponsoring organisation
Scope of the project and any specific boundaries
Constraints
Assumptions
Time-scale of the project
Deliverables and target dates (milestones)
Estimated costs
Resourcing arrangements
Reporting and monitoring arrangements
Decision-making arrangements – level of authority and accountability held by manager of project and arrangements for any necessary renegotiation
Communications arrangements
Signature of sponsor with date, title and authority

Figure 4.2 Check-list for drafting a project brief

'milestones' and these are the focus for each review period. The deliverables are the things that will be handed over or reported on at each of these review periods. For example, the full project might involve training 100 people to use new equipment within a year, but you might agree to report on progress quarterly and set targets of training 25 people in each quarter. Thus your milestones would be set as 25 trained staff each quarter. At the monitoring and review meetings you would then report on whether you had achieved this and, if there had been any slippage, how this would be recovered before the next deadline. You would also report on whether achieving the training had cost time, effort and money as estimated – whether the project was running within its budget.

It is helpful to agree the main channels of communication at this stage, whether or not they are detailed in the project brief. You need to know how to contact the key people, including the sponsor or the sponsor's delegated representative. You also need to know how they prefer to be contacted. There will be information to communicate about the progress of the projects and regular progress reports can be sent to all of those who should be kept informed. Arrangements for doing this can be agreed at the project brief stage along with any other reporting arrangements. A practical arrangement is to agree that decisions about any changes to the schedule or the resourcing can be made and signed off by the sponsor or the sponsor's representative at review meetings. You will also want to agree how to communicate if there is an urgent issue that needs immediate attention.

You might think that writing a project brief to this level of detail takes up time better spent on the project itself – but the project brief is crucial as a tool for effective management of the project. Without a brief of this type a project could progress with many successful elements, but without the overall direction and control that would ensure that it achieved its purpose. The project brief aims to establish and record agreement about the purpose, cost and timing of the project. Successful projects are all about hitting the agreed targets on time and within the agreed budget. You should now be able to prepare a project brief so that agreement can be obtained with the project sponsor. This document will provide a blueprint for the planning phase of the project.

CHAPTER 5

# MANAGING RISK

Events rarely happen in the way we expect them to, so there will always be risks associated with a project. As a project takes place in a wider environment, there are the risks normally associated with day-to-day work in that setting, including health and safety risks. There are also the risks to the project that exist only because the project exists, for example the risk that the project will not achieve its objectives.

In this chapter we consider how to identify areas of risk and what can be done to reduce the likelihood of damage to the project.

## RISK AND CONTINGENCY PLANNING

Risk is the chance that something will happen that will damage the project. Many risks can be predicted and you may feel that some aspects of risk management are simply common sense. For example, if you will not be able to start work until essential supplies are delivered, you may think of phoning the supplier to ensure that the delivery is still planned to be on time. You may also have thought well in advance and selected suppliers that you know to be reliable. However, we do not always think this carefully and some risks are not so easy to foresee.

A 'risk management' approach requires a different kind of thinking from our normal everyday approaches. It may seem rather negative and discouraging because it requires us to think about all the things that could go wrong rather than to think in positive ways about how it will look if everything flows to plan. Risk management is, however, fundamental to project management, because it enables you to plan realistically to avoid disruption by building in ways of responding to the most likely and most damaging risks if they are not preventable. As this consideration of risk informs how you plan, particularly in terms of scheduling time, effort and budgets, it needs to be done before the planning stage. Risks arise both from within the project and from the context or environment of the project.

**Example 5.1 – Internal and external risks to a project**

A hospital contracts manager was concerned about a number of complaints that had been received about the quality of cleaning. She set up a project to develop a quality monitoring system and identified some standards and performance indicators by interviewing staff in the different areas of the hospital. The cleaning contracts were due to be re-tendered and the timing was important because the new contractors would probably need to know the performance indicators when they applied to deliver the service. She was also worried about how the new standards would be monitored.

This project had a number of internal risks. There was a risk that the cleaning specifications would not be developed to reflect all of the requirements that were necessary because they had not been fully identified. There were risks associated with the rewriting of contracts and liabilities. Although the contractors are external to the hospital, concerns about the ways in which their work is carried out in the hospital are definitely part of this project and so 'internal' risks. She decided to address risks associated with rewriting contracts by working with those who won the contracts, possibly by developing performance standards during the first few months of the new contract. It might be possible to appoint a new member of staff to develop and monitor the standards, perhaps as part of a wider role.

There were no obvious external risks to this project, but some were identified when this was carefully considered. There was a risk that the hospital would not want to invest in a new member of staff or secure staff time to work on this project area. Another external risk might be that standards for cleaning might be set nationally and the hospital would then have to conform, although this project would have put it in a good position to comply with any new requirements.

In order to manage risks we need to identify them and to decide how likely it is that they will happen. It can be reassuring to consider the probability as it reduces some of the uncertainty in a project. Another way to reduce uncertainty is to consider the amount of information that is necessary in order to proceed with confidence. For example, quality is often difficult to describe in exact terms and there may be a risk that the quality of the project outcomes will not meet the expectations of the key stakeholders. This risk can be reduced by communicating with those stakeholders both before the project and as it progresses to ensure that sufficient understanding is developed and that there is time to make changes if necessary.

Consideration of risk in a project is usually limited to the possibility of different hazards impacting on the project and its purpose, not risk in any form which might affect the service or organisation in which the project is located. The only external risks that would normally be considered are those that might impact directly on the project. For example, a risk assessment for a project that involves relocating a clinic waiting room would be likely to be affected by local changes in public transport routes but a project that was developing standards for an area of service probably would not.

## PREPARING TO MANAGE RISKS

There are four stages to risk management:

1 identifying the risk – identifying what hazards are likely to affect the project and documenting the characteristics of each risk;
2 impact assessment – evaluating the risk to assess the range of possible outcomes in relation to the project and the potential impact of each of these;
3 developing plans to have in reserve to reduce the impact of the most likely risks and to ensure that these plans are implemented when necessary;
4 ensuring that the risks are kept under review and that appropriate plans are developed to meet any changes in the type or probability of adverse impact.

In many projects, these stages are considered almost simultaneously, but in large-scale projects attention should be given to each separate stage.

## CATEGORIES OF RISK

Risks arise from many different sources. These can be grouped as:

- *physical* – loss of or damage to people, equipment, stored information or buildings as a result of an accident, fire or natural disaster;
- *technical* – equipment or systems that do not work or do not work well enough to do the job intended, or that break down frequently;
- *labour* – key people unable to contribute to the project because of, for example, illness, career change or too much other work;
- *political/social* – for example, support for the project may be withdrawn as a result of a policy change by government or senior management, or because of protests from the community, the media, patients, service users or staff;
- *liability* – legal action or the threat of it because some aspect of the project is discovered to be illegal or because there may be fears of compensation claims if something goes wrong.

This list can help to identify the risks to any project. In addition, it is very helpful to discuss the project ideas with all the stakeholder groups that you can identify, because each may see the project differently and be able to identify different hazards that might be encountered.

One way to approach risk identification is not only to consider risks to the project as a whole, but also to identify risks to each of the main stages of the project. If you think of the project as a whole, risks might include the possibility of requiring some change to the key objectives. If you think of each stage, risks will be more detailed and the potential impact of hazards may change. For example, staff may be allocated to the project and may take part in the planning stage but be called to deal with unforeseen emergencies in other areas of work when they were scheduled to be implementing the project.

The whole point of identifying areas of risk is to reduce the negative impact on the project if the worst happens. If you can anticipate a risk you can prepare a plan, often called a *contingency plan*, so that you are prepared to take action to reduce the potential damage.

---

## ACTIVITY 5.1

*Allow 5 minutes.*

Imagine that you are managing a project that relies on services provided by one contractor who will work with you over a period of six months. List the possible risks associated with that contractor.

________________________________________

________________________________________

________________________________________

________________________________________

________________________________________

Your list of risks might include contractor sickness or absence, lack of promised knowledge or skills or capability. Perhaps you considered costs and whether the contractor might present higher expenses or fees than had been anticipated. You might also have noted that the contractor might work more slowly than had been scheduled.

Organisations are usually careful when contracting to include conditions about quality, time-scale and costs. However, this does not always guarantee that the service provided will be exactly what was expected and things can go wrong. It is not unusual for estimates to be insufficient for the work that needs to be done or for the time that work will take to be underestimated. In either case, there can be problems if staff have been contracted for too little time or at too low a cost.

---

## RISK ASSESSMENT AND IMPACT ANALYSIS

*Risk assessment* goes further than identifying a potential risk. To assess the risk you need to estimate how probable it is that a risk will become a reality. *Impact analysis* then builds on the assessment by considering how much damage might be caused to the project if a risk materialises.

The key questions are:

- What is the risk – how will I recognize it if it becomes a reality?
- What is the probability of it happening – high, medium or low?
- How serious a threat does it pose to the project – high, medium or low?
- What are the signals or indicators that we should be looking out for?

As you assess each risk it is usual to write them into a table, as in Table 5.1.

Table 5.1 Risk probability and impact

| | *Low impact* | *Medium impact* | *High impact* |
|---|---|---|---|
| *High probability* | | | |
| *Medium probability* | | | |
| *Low probability* | | | |

If you have identified a number of risks to assess, this table may have to be set out on a large sheet of paper or board so that you can put each risk into one of the cells. All those written into the top right-hand cell are those most dangerous to the project because they are very likely to happen and will have a very damaging impact on the project if they do happen. Others in the right-hand cells are also important to consider in your risk management planning because they have the potential to cause considerable damage although they are less likely to happen. Anything in the low impact/low probability cell can be ignored unless subsequent events lead you to reassess that risk and to place it in a higher probability category. Even then, if it will have little impact on the project you may still be able to ignore it. This is all a matter of judgement, but using a structure to organise your assessment helps to review one risk against another and to identify those for which it is important to prepare contingency plans.

## STRATEGIES FOR DEALING WITH RISK

A number of choices need to be made when considering how to manage risks. These include:

- avoiding risk – for example, you might cancel an element of a project that was in danger from a hazard that was likely to happen and would have a seriously damaging impact;
- reducing risk – for example, planning frequent reviews into the process and involving stakeholders so that they can influence progress towards acceptable outcomes;
- protecting against risk – for example, taking out insurance against particular risks;
- managing risk – for example, preparing contingency plans and revising the project plan when necessary;
- transferring risk – for example, passing responsibility for a risky task within a project to another organisation with more experience in that area of activities.

**Example 5.2 – Strategies for dealing with risk**

A personnel manager set up a pilot project to test the practicalities of an anticipated change in the law involving the employment of people with disabilities. There were questions about whether the manager was wasting money and time by running the pilot because it seemed possible that the legislation would not proceed through Parliament without substantial changes being made relating to requirements placed on employers.

The risks to this project are in the political/social category, with technical aspects. There was a risk that the project would be wasted if the anticipated change in the law did not happen or was substantially delayed. There was also a risk that the legislation would be changed and that the project would not focus on appropriate issues.

The strategy chosen was to reduce the risk. The project was slightly refocused to enable the organisation to review its current employment practices for disabled people and to make recommendations about how improvements could be made that would benefit the organisation. This provided information that enabled it to take action very quickly once the legislation details were confirmed. The organisation was able to conform with the legislative requirements while ensuring that changes that were made were of benefit to it in a number of ways.

# A CONTINGENCY PLAN

A contingency plan is one that is intended for use if a particular contingency arises. In risk management, a contingency plan is made for use if the risk becomes a reality, to minimise the damage that would be caused from its impact.

A contingency plan can be made only when risks have been identified and their probability and potential impact assessed. The purpose of the contingency plan is to limit the damage that could be inflicted on the project and to take action to move the project back into balance again. Contingency plans may include a number of different options in response to potential crisis situations. For example, you may have identified the potential risk that a flu epidemic in winter may reduce the staffing on the project during a crucial phase. One contingency plan might be to have a list of temporary staff and agencies that could be quickly approached to provide staffing if the need arose. Another contingency plan might be to delay the completion time for the project.

One perhaps less obvious advantage of creating contingency plans is that the consideration of risks can be shared with stakeholders at an early stage and potential responses discussed without the pressure of being in a crisis situation. Plans can be approved and potential costs built into reserve budgets so that action can be taken without delay if it becomes necessary.

You will need to develop contingency plans for each of the risks that you have assessed as potentially very likely to occur. Your aim should be to bring the project back on track in terms of maintaining the quality and keeping within the budget and time-scale. A risk will usually cause concern in one of the dimensions of quality, budget or time and the contingency plan will often be to increase the resource in another dimension. For example, if the risk identified is to the time-scale because one of the tasks might take much longer than estimated, the contingency plan might be to increase the budget for that task to enable more people to work on it to speed it up. If the risk is to the budget with the danger of costs escalating, the contingency might be to reduce the quality specification for some elements of the project in which the impact of quality might be less important.

## A FRAMEWORK FOR MANAGING RISK

A document called a 'risk log' or a 'risk register' is normally used to prepare a plan for management of risk. The identified risks are listed, together with the assessment of their probability and the assessment of the extent of their impact should they become a reality. Against each risk is a further column headed 'action' which outlines the contingency plan that can be put into action if the risk becomes real. An example of a risk register (or risk log) is given in Table 5.2. It provides a framework so that decisions and actions can be taken quickly when

Table 5.2 Format for a risk register

| *Risk* | *Impact* | *Probability* | *Action* |
|---|---|---|---|
| Funding | High | Low | Secure funding base prior to start of project |
| and so on with other risks | | | |

necessary. The risk register should be amended and added to regularly during the project as new risks are identified and as more is understood about the nature of risk in the project.

## INFLUENCING STAKEHOLDERS

Some projects have potential risk from stakeholders who do not fully support the aims or processes of the project. The extent of power held by stakeholders varies, but those who are powerful can be very damaging to a project and can sometimes hold the power to stop a project. You can use a technique called 'stakeholder analysis' to identify which stakeholders hold most power over the smooth progress of the project and you will then be in a position to consider how you might influence them to reduce any negative impact. Some people would consider use of this technique to be very manipulative and you will want to consider if it is appropriate to use it. In most projects it is very important to try to accommodate stakeholders' views and to respect the strength with which views are held. It is possible, however, that in some situations there are some voices that hold considerably more power than others and it might be necessary to enable weaker voices to be heard and not to be squashed by those that are loud and forceful.

Once you have identified your stakeholders and have encouraged them all to express their views about the project proposals, you can analyse stakeholder support. When you have set out the position as it appears to be from the initial views expressed, you can identify which stakeholders oppose the project or aspects of it. You can also decide where to put your efforts in influencing stakeholders to offer more support for the project or to reduce the strength of their opposition.

The first stage is to set out the stakeholders in a table as in Table 5.3 to show where you estimate their current position from the views that they have expressed. These positions are considered in terms of those who ALLOW and will not put obstacles in the way of the project, those who HELP by offering positive support and those who will try to STOP the project by whatever means they have available.

Table 5.3 Stakeholder analysis, Stage 1

| *Stakeholder* | *STOP* | *ALLOW* | *HELP* |
|---|---|---|---|
| Client | | | ✔ |
| Project team | | ✔ | |
| Other staff | ✔ | | |
| Service users | | ✔ | |
| Funders | ✔ | | |
| Media | ✔ | | |
| Voluntary organisations | | ✔ | |
| Professional bodies | | ✔ | |

Once you have mapped out these positions you can decide which of the stakeholders might be influenced to be more supportive. It is probably not worth spending time and energy trying to move stakeholders from the ALLOW position to being more positive unless you think that their help would be particularly useful. However, it is often worth trying to move those in the STOP position into ALLOW.

Table 5.4 Stakeholder analysis, Stage 2

| *Stakeholders* | *STOP* | *ALLOW* | *HELP* |
|---|---|---|---|
| Client | | | ✔ |
| Project team | | ✔ → | ? |
| Other staff | ✔ → | ? | |
| Service users | | ✔ → | ? |
| Funders | ✔ → | ? | |
| Media | ✔ → | ? | |
| Voluntary organisation | | ✔ → | ? |
| Professional bodies | | ✔ → | ? |

It is not always possible to move stakeholders from their original positions, but it is usually worth considering how fears can be reduced.

To do this you will have to focus on exactly what aspect of the project each stakeholder opposes and consider what you could do to reduce their concerns. Sometimes opposition may be because of a fear of disruption during the activities of the project. An example of this is when residents oppose project plans because they fear noise and excessive traffic. Opposition might be reduced if arrangements were made to avoid any noise at night and to put temporary road access to the site. If opinions cannot be changed then it might be necessary to take every opportunity to publicise the anticipated benefits of the project. As the project progresses and understanding develops it may become easier to change opinions.

**Example 5.3 – Managing the risks**

A voluntary organisation providing accommodation and resettlement services for homeless people proposed to extend its activities into another town where there was an established need. Local Authority financial support had been offered orally but no firm offer of funding was made in writing. Moreover, previous attempts by another organisation to do similar work met with resistance from a residents' association. Staff in the organisation were keen to support the proposal, but the manager who would be responsible for the project was on long-term sick leave.

The main risks related to staffing (labour) and to political and social factors. These issues were addressed by:

- meeting with community leaders to explain the importance and value of the new service (risk management);
- listening carefully to the concerns of the residents' association and involving them in developing more acceptable plans (influencing stakeholders);
- offering information and seeking views in the local newspaper (influencing stakeholders);
- dealing with the staff sickness problem by allocating responsibility for the new house to a different team in the interim (risk reduction);
- working with local authority staff to confirm the funding arrangements (influencing stakeholders and reducing risks);
- making sure that the draft contracts included a clause allowing the organisation to withdraw if adequate funding was not made available (risk avoidance).

Management of risk is a rather 'virtual' activity because so much of it involves anticipating hazards and imagining consequences. It brings the benefits of being well prepared for many of the predictable risks, and use of risk registers and contingency planning can save time and money when things go wrong. It can also save those managing projects a great deal of anxiety at times when things do go wrong.

CHAPTER 6

# OUTLINE PLANNING

Planning can begin once the project brief has been agreed by the project sponsors and approved by the main stakeholders. The project plan can become a working tool that helps the project team to focus on completing the project's tasks and activities. It enables those managing projects to keep track of resources, time and progress towards achieving each objective. There are many obvious benefits to thorough and careful planning, but there is a danger that energy will be put into planning and not translated into carrying out the activities of the project – planning can become an end in itself. The energy and time expended in planning needs to be in proportion to the size and complexity of the project. For most projects the time spent in defining the project brief, discussing issues with stakeholders and carrying out a risk assessment will have provided sufficient clarity to enable planning to take place. For small and fairly straightforward projects it might be sufficient to plan tasks and activities using only a few of the charts and techniques available. For larger and more complex projects there are a number of techniques that help to plan all the processes of the project so that progress can be managed and monitored.

All projects are different, so the planning for each will be different. A project is a unique activity and there is no prototype from which to predict exactly how to plan. Some of the planning and re-planning has to happen as the project work proceeds. Planning often begins during the definition phase and continues through reviews and revisions until the project is complete. In many ways it is a creative process through which you draw out an achievable way of dealing with all of the phases of the project to ensure that the objectives are achieved.

There are some basic questions to ask when you begin to plan:

- What must we do?
- When must it be done by?
- Who will do what tasks?
- What sequence will we need to do them in?
- What resources are required?

- Will this be achieved by other work not being done?
- How shall we know if it is working?

These questions can be discussed by a project team and may produce a jointly agreed plan that would be sufficient for a small and well understood project. Even then, this will probably work as a plan only if the team become committed to completing the project successfully and are willing to engage in planning and reviewing the plan. If you do hope to progress simply with the agreed answers to these questions, it is still important to write down the plan and to review it frequently to ensure that it continues to help the team to achieve the objectives.

## WHERE DO I START?

The planning stage of a project usually takes place before the activities start, but not always. In any case, planning always continues during the implementation of a project because there is always a need to change some aspects and to revise plans. It is often difficult to understand how planning relates to actions and how to keep both activities running alongside each other in a process that is working positively towards achieving the project goals.

**Example 6.1 – Linking planning and actions**

Pat was a manager in a residential home for the elderly leading a small team on a project that was intended to produce a folder of notes and protocols for common training needs, including 'moving and handling' and 'food hygiene'. The time-scale was short because the materials were needed for a planned inspection. The team were all experienced members of staff and had been enthusiastic about the project, but two months had passed and nothing had been produced.

Pat's manager, Nic, called a meeting to review progress. Pat had some notes and said that others in the team had begun to work on drafts. Nic asked for the project plan. 'I got stuck', Pat explained. 'I tried to follow the company guidelines, but I couldn't understand why we needed to produce all that paperwork because we all understood what we needed to do.' It appeared that members of the team had had different ideas about how to approach the project and had been working separately. They had not had time to meet to discuss progress. Some of them had thought that it was a good opportunity to be more creative about how things were done. Pat had felt that there was no need to produce the paperwork listed in the guidelines because time was short and they needed to get on with the work. Nic explained that the process of planning a project sets the tone for how work is done.

Pat called a meeting of the team and worked through the process with them all, so that each person understood what was needed from them. Sharing the development of the plan helped them to bring their ideas together, to agree who would do each task and to focus on how to achieve the outcomes that were required. The project was back under control and was soon completed successfully.

In Example 6.1, Pat encountered a number of barriers in planning the project. Many of these could have been overcome earlier. Pat had tried to make a plan but had found the instructions in the manual too complicated to follow. A manual of procedures was provided – but this can be bewildering for a person who does not understand why the procedures should be followed, particularly if the procedures seem to be about producing paperwork rather than carrying out the work of the project. None of the team seemed to appreciate why a plan was useful. If they had been involved in discussing the project and how they could complete it they would have realised that they needed to decide who would carry out each task and in what order these needed to be done. Involvement in planning usually also increases motivation to complete the plan. They were all feeling pressure to make progress since time was short. However, without a plan it was not clear to Pat what tasks each team member needed to do or in what order these should be done. Activity without such a plan used up energy but was frustrating since little progress with the project was achieved. A plan with targets would have helped everyone to carry out tasks that contributed to progressing the project.

The problem was identified rather late and failure would have been embarrassing for Pat and for the organisation. In this case it was not too late for corrective action to be taken to rescue the project. As this was Pat's first project, it would have been helpful for a more experienced manager to supervise Pat and to offer coaching through all of the stages of managing the project. It is possible that the culture of the organisation made it difficult to ask for support. However, if the plan had been agreed with the project sponsor there would already have been some discussion about what should be reported and when reports should be made. This would have helped to focus on whether Pat needed support before the first review date.

## DEVELOPING A PROJECT PLAN

A project plan usually includes the following elements:

- a plan of the separate tasks and activities, called a 'work breakdown structure';

- the team structure and the responsibilities of key people;
- an estimate of effort and duration for each task;
- a schedule to show the sequence and timing of activities;
- details of resources that will be allocated to each task;
- details of the budget that will be allocated to each cost that has been identified;
- contingency plans to deal with risks that have been identified.

A number of techniques and tools can help you to plan each of these elements.

You can approach planning in one of the following ways:

- Bottom up – identify all the small tasks that need to be done and then group them into larger, more manageable blocks of work.
- Top down – start by mapping out the major blocks of work that will need to be carried out and then subdivide them into their constituent tasks.
- Work backwards from the completion date if that is a given point in time, for example New Year's Day, and then fill in the intermediate stages that will enable you to get there.

Each of these approaches has advantages and disadvantages. You will need to choose the one which best fits your circumstances. Ideally, you should then use one of the other approaches to check that nothing has been missed out. It is important to record your thinking and any diagrams or charts produced since these will help to provide detail in the initial plan.

## USING A LOGIC DIAGRAM

If you want to use a bottom-up approach to planning, you can compile the activity schedule by drawing on the collective experience and knowledge of the project team that is going to carry out the tasks. Their ideas will produce a number of tasks that can be grouped into related tasks to remove any duplication. You can then start to identify activities that have to run in a sequence and those that could run concurrently. Some tasks have to be sequential because they are dependent on one another. For example, you can't put the roof on a house until you have walls strong enough to take the weight. Other tasks can run concurrently.

From the clusters of activities and tasks, you can begin to identify the project's key stages by creating a 'logic diagram'. First you have to group the activities and tasks into clusters that relate to an important milestone in the project. This will usually involve linking a number of tasks and activities that contribute to achieving something that is an important step in progressing the project. Once you have put all of the tasks and activities into groups, label them as probable key stages.

If you are not sure exactly how the clusters should be grouped and named, don't worry because you can go back and revise the groups if you realise later that some of the stages have been confused.

The next step is to sort out the order in which the key stages have to

**Example 6.2 – Key stages**

A training agency that provided work placements for young people decided to develop a directory of services available for young adults in the community. The key stages identified were:

a Secure funds
b Negotiate with other agencies
c Form advisory group
d Establish data collection plan
e Collect data
f Write directory text
g Identify printer
h Agree print contract
i Print directory
j Agree distribution plan
k Organise distribution
l Distribute directory.

Figure 6.1 shows these stages in a logic diagram. Each stage has at least one arrow entering it and one leaving: for example organising distribution (k) is dependent on agreeing a distribution plan (j) and collecting the data (e) cannot happen until a data-collection plan has been established (d). However, preparatory activities for distribution (j and k) and printing (g and h) can run concurrently. We have assumed that the advisory group will make decisions about the acceptability of the data collection and distribution plans and will agree the printing contract.

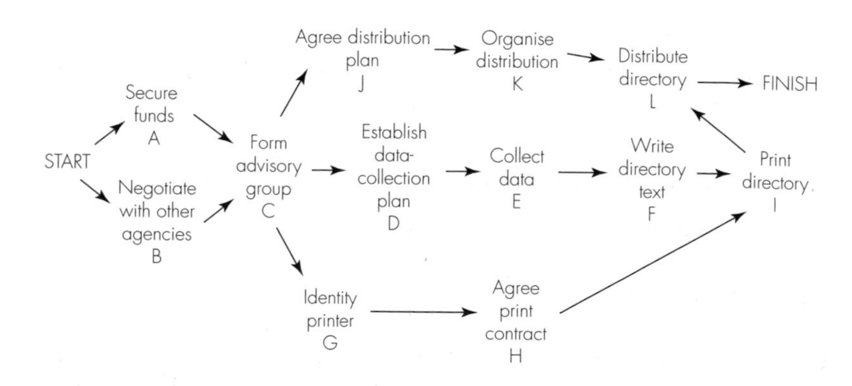


Figure 6.1 Logic diagram for directory production

be carried out to complete the objectives of the project. This exercise can be approached by writing the key stages on cards or coloured self-adhesive notes, so that you can move the notes around and then arrange them on a whiteboard or a large sheet of paper. Put cards labelled 'start' and 'finish' on the board first and then arrange the key stages between them in the appropriate sequence. Then draw arrows to link the stages in a logical sequence, taking care to consider the order in which the key stages have to be carried out. The arrows indicate that each stage is dependent on another. This means that the second stage cannot be started until the first is completed. The idea of 'dependency' is important in managing projects because if you don't work out the stages that must be completed first, people can be waiting around and wasting time until an essential earlier stage is finished before it is possible to start the next stage.

When you draw a logic diagram the following conventions may be helpful:

- Time flows from 'Start' on the left to 'Finish' on the right, but there is no limited time-scale.
- Each key stage must be described separately. If you find that you have missed one out you can add it and rearrange the others if you plan your diagram with cards before drawing out the finished picture.
- The duration of key stages is not relevant yet because you do not have to work within a fixed time-scale at this stage of planning.
- Different coloured cards can be used for different kinds of activities.
- Take time to debate and agree the place of each card in the diagram.
- Once you are fairly sure of the layout, show the dependency links with arrows.
- When your diagram is complete, try working backwards to check whether it will work. Make sure that the project achieves all of its objectives.
- Don't assign tasks to people yet.
- Keep a record once the diagram has been agreed, copying out the positions of key stages and the dependency arrows.

## ACTIVITY 6.1

*Allow 30 minutes.*

Imagine that managers in your organisation are considering developing a directory to be given to new staff appointed, as part of the induction process. You expect that you will be asked to manage this project. You want to be well prepared for the meeting at which the potential project will be discussed. Draw up a list of the tasks involved in the project and organise them into key stages as a logic diagram.

Feedback: Your diagram probably looked similar to the one in Figure 6.1. You should have noted that you would need approval to use resources (A), which might include approval to involve others in the organisation and to interview people in each area of work (B). You might have decided to have some sort of steering committee (C) – this is often a good idea because it brings ideas from various perspectives to the project and it also helps to attract support for the project and its outcomes. You would have needed to plan for data collection (D and E) and someone would have to create the text (F) which would need to be printed or produced in an accessible electronic form (I) so that new people to the organisation could easily access the information. The production process would need steps G and H, as in the earlier logic diagram. You would also need to consider how the directory should be distributed to each area of work in the organisation (J, K and L). There are essentially three sequences of activities that must be completed in sequential order before the whole project can be completed.

---

In general, once you have an overview of the key activities and stages of the project, you have the skeleton of your plan. You can then work out the details in each of the stages. However, the plan will not be static and the world will not stop while you develop your plan. While planning takes place, other events are changing the situations that surround the project. Your understanding of the project will develop and change as you become more familiar with the issues raised in each stage of planning.

Planning is a dynamic process and one of your main roles in managing a project is to keep the balance between:

- the need to have a plan to ensure that the project outcomes can be achieved within time, budget and quality requirements, and
- the need to respond to changes in the setting surrounding the project and in the understanding of all of the people involved in the project.

In some ways the plan is like an idealised picture of what should happen and you use it to help to keep the project on track while things inevitably change around you.

It is helpful to keep the project brief as the starting point in each stage of planning, to ensure that the purpose of the project is not forgotten in the practicalities of planning. As each part of the plan develops, use the project brief as a basis for checking that the key outcomes are still the focus of activity and that the balance of budget, schedule and quality are being maintained.

## IDENTIFYING DELIVERABLES

The term 'deliverables' is used to describe everything that is to be produced and handed over during the project – everything that has to be delivered. It is important to identify the deliverables because these provide a focus to help you to be sure that the project is planned to achieve all of the things expected of it.

The project brief will identify the goals of the project and may express some of these as key objectives. There will be other objectives that may be supplementary to the key objectives. Some of the objectives will be explicit about what is to be produced. Others may detail an outcome that cannot be achieved without the completion of some preliminary steps and these can be identified as implicit in the objective. At an early stage of planning you will need to identify all of the project objectives and the deliverables that are implied or explicitly required from each objective.

Each objective will identify a clear outcome. The outcome is the deliverable. In some cases, the outcome will be some sort of change achieved and in other cases it will be the production of something new. In either case, the deliverable should be identified so that it will be easy to demonstrate that it has been achieved. For example, the first objective in a project that aimed to change the service focus of an organisation was to ensure that all of the key managers were trained to carry out the change. The deliverable might have been evidence that 80 key managers had been trained in managing change. This evidence might have taken the form of records showing that the training had taken place. If the training really was the objective, then this would be sufficient. However, the training was intended as preparation for action. It might have been closer to the purpose of this project if the deliverable for this objective had been framed in terms of each of the 80 trained managers being able to provide evidence of having successfully managed change.

Even this deliverable would not, in itself, support the project manager's personal intention to raise the profile of the human resources department within the organisation. To achieve this, he might have decided to collect evidence that these 80 managers had successfully managed change and then used this evidence to produce a report as the deliverable. This would show how the training provided by the HR department had succeeded in developing these managers so that they were able to contribute effectively to organisational change. It is important to ensure that the outcomes of the project are the ones intended and this can be focused with specific objectives and identified deliverables.

The definition of outputs and outcomes is difficult. Outputs can be defined when there is a distinctly identifiable product, but outcomes are more holistic and can imply a changed state that might not be evident for some time. In some situations it is particularly difficult, where cause and effect are uncertain or where there are conflicts of values. It is still important in such settings to identify goals and to define them in a way that will enable an appraisal of the extent to which the aims of the project have been achieved. This does not necessarily mean that quantitative measures should be imposed, because inappropriate use of measures can lead to goal displacement. It can be helpful to ask, 'How shall we know if we have been successful?' and identify the indicators that will help in making that judgement.

**Example 6.3 – Deliverables**

The training agency directory of services had a series of objectives that had enabled them to identify the key stages given in Example 6.2. The initial list of deliverables drawn up by the project manager included notes about how each deliverable could be demonstrated as successfully achieved.

a – Secure funds
Deliverables are:

- funding available to be used when necessary (demonstrated by authority agreed to sign cheques);
- budget statement prepared with headings identifying key areas of expenditure;
- agreement with sponsor about how expenditure will be recorded and how orders, invoices and receipts will be managed.

b – Negotiate with other agencies
Deliverables are:

- notes and minutes of formal meetings with potential collaborators identifying comments about the project and issues raised;
- signed agreements recording formal agreements about funding or sharing of information or records;
- nominations of staff to serve on the advisory group (list of names with organisation and contact details).

c – Form advisory group
Deliverables are:

- membership list indicating organisations represented;
- schedule of planned meetings;
- written terms of reference for the group focusing on achieving the project outcomes and accommodating any concerns raised during negotiations;
- plan to show how the advisory group will inform and advise the progress of the project.

d – Establish data collection plan
Deliverables are:

- written plan describing what data will be collected from whom, when and in what form. Decision necessary about how to collate before data is collected as this will influence whether we collect in electronic or paper-based form. Need to check compatability of systems and gain agreement about form.

e – Collect data
Deliverables are:
- data collected according to agreed plan;
- data collated in a way that enables directory text to be written.

f – Write directory text
Deliverables are:
- staff to write contracted or released with time to do it;
- written agreement about the anticipated size and contents of the document;
- agreement about how logos will be used;
- full information available from data collection and collation;
- draft directory text written and distributed to agencies or advisory group for comment;
- finished written directory text.

g – Identify printer
Deliverables are:
- agreement about a process for selection of a printer;
- documents inviting printers to tender or estimate;
- agreement about criteria for selection of an appropriate printer;
- at least three estimates from printers;
- completion of process of selection and printer identified.

h – Agree print contract
Deliverables are:
- contract written;
- contract agreed with printer and signed.

i – Print directory
Deliverables are:
- agreed number of directories printed to the quality agreed, by the date agreed and delivered for storing as agreed.

j – Agree distribution plan
Deliverables are:
- written plan for distribution agreed with all other agencies.

k – Organise distribution
Deliverables are:
- plan for distribution identifies who should do what to ensure distribution as agreed.

l – Distribute directory
Deliverables are:
- directories are received in all locations agreed.

The project manager realised that the process of thinking through all of the deliverables raised many more issues than had been fully discussed when the project brief was agreed. For example, all of the activity focused on achieving the distribution of the directory, but they had not discussed how they would evaluate the usefulness of the directory when it was available for use in these locations. They also had not discussed how it might be updated – but there was an opportunity to do that when deciding what form it should be in. They had not really discussed whether the whole thing might be better developed as a website and if they did that, they would not need printers but they would need web designers and some way of managing the site. In many ways, working through the details of the project in this way brought out aspects of the project that needed to be considered before progressing much further. Sometimes it is not until you begin to imagine the deliverables that you can see whether the purpose of the project will be achieved in the way originally proposed.

One more aspect of deliverables is that they need to be handed over to someone authorised to receive them. The handover procedures need to be agreed with the sponsor so that as each deliverable is handed over there is a formal acknowledgement that the specification has been fully met. A record is usually kept to show that each item has been 'signed off' as fully acceptable.

In some cases, users will need some training to be able to use or implement the deliverable. It is important to agree who will be responsible for the ongoing training or implementation, so that there are no misunderstandings about the boundary of the project. If the identification of a deliverable raises issues of this nature, the project manager might find that a new element is added to the project as a new objective and deliverable in the form of a training or implementation plan. This would, of course, also necessitate consideration of the schedule and budget to ensure that this additional new element could be delivered within the existing agreements or whether an additional allowance must be made.

Once you have a logic diagram showing the order in which the key stages of the project should be carried out and a list of deliverables, you can check each of these against the other to make sure that you have included everything in the key stages. These provide the basics of a project plan. What is still missing is a schedule for the key stages and the tasks and activities within them that will ensure that the project is completed within the time-scale allowed. There is not yet a detailed estimate of how long each task or activity might take or how much it will cost, so neither time-scale nor budget can be managed in detail. Although the deliverables have been identified, there may be different perceptions about what level of quality is acceptable and this may need to be detailed more carefully. This level of outline planning may be sufficient for uncomplicated projects where the team knows the issues very well, but most projects will require further planning to enable management in more detail.

CHAPTER 7

# ESTIMATING TIME AND COSTS

Estimating is crucial to planning. Before you can plan how to complete tasks and activities, you need to have some idea of how long each will take and what resources will be needed to complete it. If you know that one task has to be completed before another can be started, you need to know how long the first task will take before you can schedule when the second task can start. When you have to consider contracting and paying staff to carry out particular tasks, substantial costs can be involved and considerable waste if the estimates are inaccurate. To some extent, estimating is always a guess. As in most guessing, your judgement can be improved by knowledge and experience (whether this is your own or that of those you consult) and by use of some of the tools and techniques that can support decision-making.

## ESTIMATING TIME

Many people find it very difficult to estimate how long a task or key stage in a project will take to complete. You might approach the problem in a number of ways:

- consider the size and complexity of each task and how much time you would allow if it was part of a day-to-day workload;
- consult someone who is experienced in carrying out similar tasks;
- review previous projects where a similar task has been completed.

Another way would be to start from the amount of time that you want to allow for the task and work out how many people would be needed to complete it in the time available.

Where a project has a fixed end-date (for example an event where a celebrity will declare a new building open) there is a natural tendency to try to compress the schedule to fit all the key stages into the time available. All too often it becomes clear later that the schedule is impossible. It is better to be realistic at the outset and be clear about what can be delivered and what cannot. Productive time may only amount to 3.5 to 4 days per week and time needs to be built in for meetings, communication, co-ordination and line-management arrangements. You will also need to allow some extra time for contingencies such as unexpected interruptions that cannot be predicted.

The objectives will have identified what is to be achieved and when it should be completed. The objective-setting process should also have tried to ensure that each objective is manageable, measurable and achievable, or at least considered the extent to which these conditions could be met. Each objective can be divided further to identify the steps that must be taken to complete the objective and the tasks that will contribute to achieving the outcome. As in all planning, this process is continuous. As new information becomes available and as the project progresses, changes will need to be made to aspects of the objectives and to the sequences of tasks that contribute to achievement of the completed project.

## WORK BREAKDOWN STRUCTURE

As a starting point, it is usual to divide the work of a project into tasks that enable you to identify project staff for each aspect of the work to be carried out. A *work breakdown structure* enables you to divide the work of a project into 'packages'. These can be further subdivided into 'elements' and then into individual tasks that provide a basis for estimating the time and effort required.

The first stage in starting to draw up a work breakdown structure is to divide the project into its main parts. These are quite high-level descriptions of the work of the project. For example, if the project purpose is to relocate a service delivery area the main areas to start the work breakdown would probably be:

- prepare for the move;
- carry out the move;
- re-establish the service provision.

The next step is to divide each of these into the main activities that will contribute to achieving each outcome. For example, to prepare for the move there would be an area of activity that made arrangements with service users and anyone else who would be affected to temporarily suspend the service and an area that was concerned with packing equipment and materials. To continue the breakdown, each of these would be further detailed until lists of distinct tasks had been identified.

The work breakdown structure identifies and defines each of the project tasks in considerable detail. Once each task has been identified, consideration can be given to planning how it will be completed. For each task there are a number of questions to consider:

- What skills and experience are required to complete the task?
- What materials are required to complete the task?
- What equipment, conditions or information are required to complete the task?
- How much time will be required to complete the task?

It is usually advisable to involve the project team in constructing the work breakdown structure as it can be one of the initial team-building tasks and can provide the first opportunity to develop an understanding of the whole project. A full team discussion can help to minimise duplication of tasks.

This information should be recorded so that if a problem arises that threatens completion of any task, the project manager can consider how to address the problem. For example, if the team member who was to complete the task falls ill, the need for skills and experience can be reviewed and a suitable substitute sought.

In a large project, the work breakdown structure might allow packages of work to be allocated to teams or team members so that they could identify and schedule the sub-tasks. It is important to identify each deliverable in the work breakdown structure so that all the activities can be seen to contribute towards achieving the deliverables.

**Example 7.1 – Part of the work breakdown structure for establishing a new clinic**

The purpose of the project was to convert a large room connected to a Primary Care reception area into a new clinic to treat minor injuries. The work had been broken down into two packages, building work and service preparation. A package of work is a group of related activities and tasks that can be conveniently considered together. It is not necessary for them to be grouped under different team responsibilities, but this can be a useful method for identifying the package of work for a team. This method can also be used to identify costs related to each package of work or drawn up to identify the wider resource requirements. It is simply a way of dividing the whole project into manageable parts so that the implications can be considered and progress planned.

Each package was broken down into a list of activities that would have to be completed. Work breakdown structure does not include scheduling, so there was no need at this stage to consider the sequence of activities. Each activity was then divided into separate tasks (see Table 7.1).

Table 7.1 shows the work breakdown structure as it looked when the first two sets of tasks had been identified. This level of detail then had to be completed for the tasks in each activity.

It is very useful to try to identify each activity and task in terms of the outcome or deliverable for each item, as this will then provide an overall list of deliverables. In some cases there will be several deliverables from each item in the activities list. The work associated with achieving each deliverable is probably a separate task.

Table 7.1 Work breakdown structure for new minor injury clinic

| *Packages* | *Building work* | *Service preparation* |
|---|---|---|
| *Activities* | 1. survey site<br>2. plan alterations<br>3. estimate building work<br>4. contract builders<br>5. purchase equipment and materials<br>6. carry out building work | 1. plan service provision<br>2. inform potential service users<br>3. estimate resources needed<br>4. secure staff and prepare rotas<br>5. purchase equipment and materials<br>6. prepare for service delivery |
| *Tasks* | *Activity 1: survey site*<br>contract surveyor<br>prepare list of alterations<br>identify any problems or opportunities<br>revise list<br><br>*Activity 2: plan alterations*<br>plan layout and partitions<br>plan access<br>plan work areas<br>plan electric points<br>plan lighting<br>plan flooring<br>plan storage<br>plan decorations<br>draw up specifications | |

As the work breakdown is considered, groups of activities might be identified that could be considered as mini-projects in themselves. These can be treated as such and could offer useful staff development opportunities for team leaders in appropriate areas of work. It can be attractive to the team and sponsor to use the opportunity of a project to provide staff development, but the purpose and deliverables of the project have to be considered carefully so that there is no diversion from the purpose. If substantial staff development is intended, this should appear as an objective and deliverables identified so that the project is focused appropriately.

**Example 7.2 – Developing the work breakdown structure with the team**

An experienced project manager said that he always holds a brainstorming session with his project team as part of a workshop to develop a shared understanding about the project. 'This workshop is often the first opportunity for the team to work together. I encourage everyone to contribute their ideas about the project and the various tasks. During the workshop I begin to allocate responsibility for tasks when it is appropriate for particular individuals to lead them so that they can shape the approach from the start.

'It is great to see people becoming enthusiastic and wanting to get on with organising each task, but there is a danger at this stage. I sometimes find that people with expertise and experience want to plan things in a way that demonstrates and possibly develops their areas of interest rather than focusing on achieving what the project needs. I avoid letting things get out of hand by putting up the project deliverables before sorting out who will lead in each area, so that the whole team stay focused on what we are trying to achieve rather than what role they will take. I try to make sure that all the "experts" commit to supporting achievement of all the deliverables so that they collaborate to help others complete their tasks as well as working on their own. It doesn't always work because of personalities, but at least it usually sets the "tone" of the project and emphasises that teamwork matters.'

This approach also gives the project manager confidence that the project has been thought through properly so that all the deliverables are achievable.

## STAFF COSTS

Once the work breakdown plan is complete it becomes possible to cost the project. There is usually a balance to achieve between the overall figure that has been identified as a budget for the project and the costs that can be identified once the detailed planning has begun. If you are confident that the tasks are realistic and can be achieved, you can begin to estimate the cost of staff time. There will be other staff-related costs if the project is to employ staff directly, for example costs of administration of salaries, taxation, holiday allowances, overtime payments, training, travel and subsistence. There may also be accommodation costs for staff and equipment for the duration of the project.

In some cases it is less costly for an organisation to hire staff specifically to work on a project than to redeploy existing staff. This is particularly likely if existing staff would have to be trained before they could carry out the project tasks. This raises the question of whether the organisation might want to train its existing staff (if the skills will be necessary in future) or whether hiring the necessary skills for the period of the project might be the most appropriate approach. If training existing staff becomes a preferred choice, this needs to be written into the objectives of the project and the costs and staffing associated with training become another key stage to incorporate.

Staff costs for a project can be estimated by analysing the project into tasks and working out staff requirements in terms of the skills and experience required and the number of staff that will be needed to complete the tasks within the time-scale available. Appropriate rates of pay can then be decided. Organisations that use project approaches in much of their work often have standard approaches to calculating and costing staff time. Some organisations use formulas to calculate costs. These formulas include ratios of staff to clients (for example the number of clients in a social worker's workload) and of one staff group to another (for example the ratio of clinical staff to administrative staff).

## AVOIDING ABUSIVE PRACTICES

When a project is set up without consideration of the potential impact of redirecting staff from their usual work to the project, all sorts of questions are raised. The basic assumptions about staff and accommodation availability need to be discussed at an early stage because this can make a lot of difference to the costs that are identified. Assumptions about the extent to which staff can be asked to work on projects that differ from their normal employment conditions can also be an issue if people are not employed for flexible working. It is often tempting not to formalise these issues if project working can be 'hidden' in an organisation budget because only part of the time of individual members of staff is to be used. However, this opens the door to potential abuse of those individuals if they are asked to work on projects and to continue to deliver all of their usual work outcomes. When several managers share claims on the time of a member of staff there can be pressure to achieve performance levels in several different areas of work with no mechanism for overseeing the workload of the individual.

Many health and social care organisations are moving towards increasing use of project working because it is seen as beneficial in identifying focused outcomes for areas of work. It is, however, unusual for the time involved in developing project proposals to be identified as an activity separate from normal day-to-day work although this is additional work unless the workloads are adjusted to accommodate this responsibility. Projects are often set up in a work area where individuals already have a full workload with the expectation that everyone will take part in the project without additional resources. This enables the project outcomes to be achieved without identifying a special budget for the work. This is not, in itself, a problem if the organisation approves of the practice, but staff members need to be protected from abuse by careful management of workloads. In many organisations it is possible to refocus work for a period of time to enable small projects to be completed. If project working is to take place in this way, organisations need to develop mechanisms to manage variations in workloads to maintain fair working practices. It is not quick or easy to change the employment practices of an organisation to accommodate flexible working.

There is a danger in not costing the staffing of a project. There may be a cost to the organisation of the staff not being available to carry out the day-to-day core work for which they were employed. If the project staffing costs are not estimated, the cost of the project is not formally considered. If the organisation is to invest staff time, there should be some discussion about whether the value of the outcomes of the project justifies that expenditure. Sometimes such a discussion is avoided because those who want to carry out the project are worried that others will not recognise the value as worth the cost. This can be a problem in an organisation that is reluctant to encourage innovation.

**Example 7.3 – Workload problems**

A small charity that worked with distressed children in the community recognised that their workers were finding work increasingly stressful. When a child or family requested help they responded by making appointments for face-to-face meetings as soon as possible. Everyone was frustrated that increasing workloads had led to appointments with new clients being delayed so that many feared that situations would worsen to danger levels. Funding was always insufficient and the flow of funding unreliable, so the appointment of additional staff was impossible.

In an attempt to improve working lives, staff had developed a number of projects that they had shared responsibility for completing. These included the development of better appointment scheduling, changing the use of some of the rooms to provide more appointment rooms and increasing the range of work that could be carried out by unqualified volunteers. Although everyone supported the intentions of these projects and wanted to complete them, agreeing to take a role in the projects had increased the stress felt by many staff. Frustration was increased because few found time to make any progress at all towards achieving the project outcomes.

The situation did not improve until some more strategic thinking took place among the senior staff and the charity Management Board. They decided to form partnerships with other local voluntary organisations and the statutory Social Services to refer clients who could be supported in the long term by these other organisations. This changed the role of the charity to some extent, in that it acted more as an emergency resource and a short-term support. They took the opportunity to review their conditions of employment to build project working into the job descriptions. They also revised their line management arrangements to ensure that individual workloads could be managed flexibly.

In health and social care there is a great emphasis on carrying out projects to support major changes intended to modernise services. In many organisations there is an urgent need to review and revise workload allocation to ensure that staff are treated fairly. In under-funded services there is often reluctance to identify the full staff costs of projects that are intended to improve service provision. Where staff are struggling to achieve project outcomes alongside responsibility for providing services to vulnerable or injured people, the stress involved in trying to do a good job can be very damaging.

## EQUIPMENT COSTS

Unless the project is to be housed in accommodation normally used for different purposes, there will be costs associated with providing telephones and computers. If the project is to make temporary use of accommodation, the project activities will require funding and some equipment will normally be needed.

Most organisations make a distinction between costs that relate to buying something that will be a long-term asset, which would normally be considered as capital expenditure, and expenses that are not related to a significant purchase. The work breakdown plan will give information about what equipment and materials will be required for each task and the costs of these can be investigated and estimated.

If the organisation already has whatever equipment is needed, the only costs relating to the project may be those associated with redeploying the equipment for temporary use on the project, including any loss of value through wear and tear. However, if equipment is normally in use elsewhere, an opportunity cost will be incurred in taking it away from its normal use. For example, a unit needed an additional fax machine for two months and borrowed one from their research unit, where it was used for routine but non-urgent communications. However, the research unit found that many of its usual communications were badly disrupted during this period because people had become used to using the fax. The greatest problem was that many of their colleagues travelling in India, Australia and New Zealand had great difficulty in telephoning the office because of the time zone differences. The loss of the fax machine, even for a short period, proved to be expensive in the time spent compensating for its absence.

If the organisation does not already have the necessary equipment, or cannot spare it from elsewhere for temporary use on the project, it may be bought or hired. This raises similar considerations to those relating to whether to hire new staff or train existing staff. If one of the project objectives is to purchase new equipment and to train staff to use it confidently, then identifying suitable equipment and purchasing it will be entirely appropriate. If this is not so, it may be more appropriate to hire it for the length of time that it is needed.

Equipment costs are not limited to acquisition costs. Most equipment needs regular maintenance, it will break down and need repairing, it will require fuel or energy, and it will need accommodation or garaging and security. All these costs of keeping and operating equipment should be considered. And someone will probably be needed to use the equipment. This might entail costs relating to skilled use of equipment and supervision and training for staff unfamiliar with the equipment.

## MATERIALS COSTS

Many categories of materials, supplies and consumables will be used in a project. Once again, the materials that are in constant use and easily and 'freely' available in an organisation might be overlooked in costing the project. For example, it is easy to assume that stationery will be available in much the same way as it is for day-to-day work. However, a project is a bounded activity, and if you are to understand the full cost of achieving the outcomes, you will need to know how much the whole range of activity costs. For example, a project can easily and inconspicuously increase the organisation's operating costs of postage and telephone or of paper and printing.

If the project involves constructing something from materials, there will be a cost related to raw materials. This may include costs for transport and storage if the materials have to be moved to the site at which they will be used and stored safely. Materials that are fragile or which have a limited life will need special consideration. For example, if the purpose of the project is to stage an event at which food will be served, the timing and storage considerations will be very different from projects that involve use of materials that will last indefinitely.

## ESTIMATING REVENUES AND INTANGIBLE BENEFITS

If one of your project outcomes involves increasing revenue, there are some particular considerations in estimating the level of income that might be expected. If the costs of the project are to be recovered by sales, then the price of products must reflect not only the costs of the project but also the costs of adminstration required to collect the sales income.

Pricing is a complicated business. If the project involves developing products for sale, it is usually necessary to carry out some market research to ensure that the products will be welcome and that people will be willing to pay for them. Prices are usually set to enable costs to be covered and some profit to be made, but prices also have to relate to the prices charged for similar products that are available. For example, if your project aimed to develop a book support stand and light for wheelchair users, you would have to check that people did want to read while in their wheelchairs and that they would prefer to read books and not newspapers or magazines. You might also investigate whether people intended to make use of hand-held readers for electronic books.

A product that is intended to produce revenue has to be something that people will want to buy at the price you want to charge. We are usually advised to estimate costs on the high side and potential revenues on the low side to build in some safety in case estimates are not very accurate.

## WHO SHOULD ESTIMATE?

The person managing the project is not necessarily the best one to prepare the estimates, although they should be closely involved because they need a clear understanding of what the estimates assume about the project. If there are others who have more experience or more knowledge about some of the areas of work, these people may be the best ones to make estimates for the project or parts of it. You could ask each person to work independently and then hold a meeting to compare estimates and to discuss how to arrive at realistic figures.

If someone associated with the project has experience of estimating, it could be very valuable to involve them. It is also often helpful to take advice about any risks relating to the areas of revenues and costs. For example, if you will need to buy materials, the prices of raw materials might vary over time or according to the quantity of the order. In a large project, the services of an experienced buyer might contribute cost savings.

## PLANNING FOR QUALITY

Having considered estimating for time and for costs, remember that the project cannot succeed unless the outcomes are of an appropriate quality. There is often a tendency to reduce the time allowed to complete tasks and activities if estimates of cost are higher than expected. The need to achieve a particular level of quality may mean that more time must be spent completing one or another task or that more resources must be made available for a particular purpose. Once the time and cost estimates have been made, review them to ensure that this estimate will allow an outcome of the right quality.

If insufficient information is available to make this calculation, it might be possible to carry out a small part of one task to give a little more information about the practical realities. If the project involves staff in carrying out unfamiliar tasks, training might be needed. If training is required, it might be important to consider how quickly staff will be able to carry out the task once they are confident and experienced – and how long it will take for them to reach this level of competence.

Many organisations have corporate quality assurance systems that have to be applied to any project for which they are responsible. However, difficulties may arise when several quality assurance systems are in operation in a multi-agency project. In such a case, it would be possible to include the development of an appropriate quality assurance framework as part of the project itself, so that the project sponsors and stakeholders are fully included in the processes that deliver outcomes to them.

Quality assurance procedures should be set up as early as possible in a project's life cycle, so that appropriate systems can be put in place and the procedures for monitoring can be communicated throughout the project system. If the project is large or complex, part of the documentation may include a 'quality manual' which describes the aims of the project, how each part of the project system is organised functionally, procedural documentation that states how each task is to be completed, and any relevant technical specifications. As in any other area of planning, this would not be appropriate for a small project and care should be taken not to spend time, energy and resources on the production of anything that does not contribute directly to the achievement of the project outcomes.

CHAPTER 8

# SCHEDULING

Projects consist of a number of tasks and activities and one of the key planning issues is to decide how long each will take to complete and the order in which these should take place. It is not enough to decide how long each individual task will take, because some tasks cannot be started until others are completed. Scheduling involves decisions about timing and sequence. The full costs of a project, both in financial terms and in staffing effort, cannot be estimated until the time to complete the full project outcomes is identified.

## TIMING AND SEQUENCE

A rough estimate might be made based on previous experience of a similar project, but a clearer picture can be obtained by making the calculations necessary to schedule a project. To do this, each task has to be estimated in terms of the content of the work, the number of staff that will be needed to complete it and the overall time that the task will take. This will allow you to work out the resources required. You can schedule by taking into account the current workloads of the project team members, which might affect the start date, and their capacity to carry out the work. This brings you into the detail of deciding whether additional staff will be necessary or whether the project tasks should be scheduled to enable work already committed to be completed first.

In most projects, some tasks form the foundations for others and thus have to be completed first. For example, floors have to be laid before carpets or other surfaces can be put onto them. This is called *dependency*. One task is dependent on another being completed before it can begin. Dependency is very important in planning a project because it can be very costly if staff time is wasted because they are available but not able to start work until others have completed their tasks. There is also the possibility of delay if estimates prove to be wrong about how long the earlier tasks will take.

Two techniques will help in planning timing and sequence. The Gantt chart enables you to block out periods of time to gain an overview of the project tasks and the time-scale to completion. This is an easy technique to use and quickly gives a picture of the main sequence that will necessary. The Gantt chart is not so useful for identifying the detail of dependencies or the potential impact of a delay in the sequence of tasks. A technique called Critical Path Analysis (CPA) is frequently used to schedule tasks and to identify the potential implications of each dependency.

## DRAWING UP A GANTT CHART

A Gantt chart shows the key stages of a project and the duration of each as a bar chart. The time-scale runs across the top and the tasks are listed on the left-hand side, in sequence from the first task. The bars are shaded to show how long each key task will take. The bar for the last task finishes in the bottom right-hand corner to show when the project will be completed. Figure 8.1 shows the first Gantt chart for a project for determining the need for a new clinical assessment technique within a community mental health environment, showing bar lines for the main objectives. A Gantt chart can be drawn quickly and easily and is often done at an early stage to gain an overview of the time that the whole project will take to complete. It is easy to see if the project will take longer to complete than expected and whether the initial plans are achievable. A more detailed Gantt chart is usually completed once the main objectives have been determined.

For a complex project you may decide to produce a separate Gantt chart for each of the key stages. If you do this shortly before each key stage begins, you will be able to take any last-minute eventualities into account. These charts provide a useful tool for monitoring and control as the project progresses.

You can add other information to a Gantt chart, for example:

- Milestones – you might prefer to indicate these with a symbol such as a triangle;
- Project meetings – these might be indicated with a different symbol such as a circle;
- Key review dates.

## USING COMPUTER PROGRAMS TO PLAN AND SCHEDULE

Gantt charts are relatively easy to draw by hand, but this doesn't offer you the same level of flexibility during monitoring that you would get from a software package. Various programs are available to assist project managers in scheduling and control. Moreover, once the data have been entered, a program helps you to work on 'what if' scenarios, showing what might happen if a key stage is delayed or speeded up. This is more difficult if you are working manually. Computer software also allows you to move easily from one level of detail to another.

A number of different software packages are designed to help you to produce a project plan. These are often quite powerful and complex

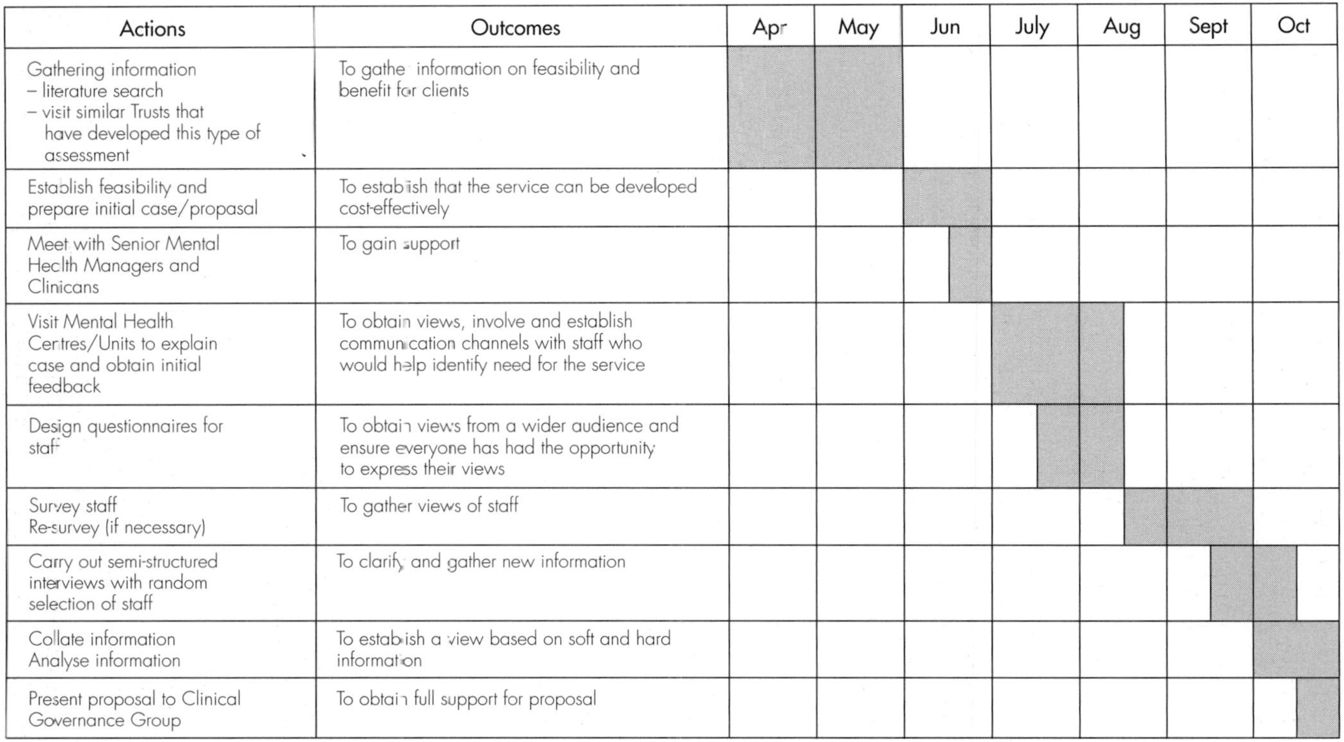

| Actions | Outcomes | Apr | May | Jun | July | Aug | Sept | Oct |
|---|---|---|---|---|---|---|---|---|
| Gathering information<br>– literature search<br>– visit similar Trusts that have developed this type of assessment | To gather information on feasibility and benefit for clients | | | | | | | |
| Establish feasibility and prepare initial case/proposal | To establish that the service can be developed cost-effectively | | | | | | | |
| Meet with Senior Mental Health Managers and Clinicans | To gain support | | | | | | | |
| Visit Mental Health Centres/Units to explain case and obtain initial feedback | To obtain views, involve and establish communication channels with staff who would help identify need for the service | | | | | | | |
| Design questionnaires for staff | To obtain views from a wider audience and ensure everyone has had the opportunity to express their views | | | | | | | |
| Survey staff<br>Re-survey (if necessary) | To gather views of staff | | | | | | | |
| Carry out semi-structured interviews with random selection of staff | To clarify and gather new information | | | | | | | |
| Collate information<br>Analyse information | To establish a view based on soft and hard information | | | | | | | |
| Present proposal to Clinical Governance Group | To obtain full support for proposal | | | | | | | |

Figure 8.1 A Gantt chart for determining the need for a new clinical assessment technique within a community mental health environment

*Source*: Stephen Oliver, Management Training Consultant, Business Development Consultancy

and it may take some time to learn to use them. At the early stages of a project, people often start the planning on paper or use a simple program, perhaps a spread-sheet. Once the outline plans have been made, computer programs provide a very flexible way of managing the project if you have learnt to use them. For those whose work will often include project management it is a good idea to develop skills and familiarity with some of the available software. Some organisations use a project management protocol for all of their projects to ensure that there is a similar approach to project management and to enable a central record of projects to be available to managers.

## IDENTIFYING THE CRITICAL PATH

The critical path is the sequence of tasks that will enable the project to be completed in the shortest possible time. It identifies which tasks must be completed before others can follow. Identification of the critical path is important in projects that must be completed in the shortest possible time. It is also important when the costs of running a project are significant because careful scheduling can ensure that the least number of days possible are spent carrying out the project.

To identify the critical path, the length of time that each task will take has to be calculated. Then the dependencies have to be identified. There may be dependencies in each of the different sequences of activity that contribute to completion of the project. The work breakdown structure is usually the starting point as this will identify the packages of activities and the individual tasks.

**Example 8.1 – Part of the work breakdown structure for relocation of an office**

**Packages of activities**

| **1. Prepare the site** | **2. Furnish and equip office** | **3. Service preparation** |
|---|---|---|
| 1.1 survey site | 2.1 plan furnishing needs | 3.1 plan service during the move |
| 1.2 plan alterations | 2.2 identify what we have | 3.2 inform potential service users |
| 1.3 estimate building work | 2.3 purchase furniture | 3.3 arrange resources needed |
| 1.4 contract builders | 2.4 plan equipment needs | 3.4 deliver service during move |
| 1.5 purchase building materials | 2.5 identify what we have | 3.5 prepare staff locations and rotas |
| 1.6 carry out building | 2.6 purchase equipment | 3.6 prepare info about new location |
| | 2.7 install furniture | 3.7 inform when move completed |
| | 2.8 install equipment and connect | |

**Activities divided into tasks**

**Activity 1.1: survey site**

1.1.1 contract surveyor
1.1.2 prepare list of alterations
1.1.3 identify any problems or opportunities
1.1.4 revise list

**Activity 1.2: plan alterations**

1.2.1 plan layout and partitions
1.2.2 plan access
1.2.3 plan work areas
1.2.4 plan electric points
1.2.5 plan lighting
1.2.5 plan flooring
1.2.6 plan storage
1.2.7 plan decorations
1.2.8 draw up specifications

(This will be continued until each activity is divided into tasks.)

The full work breakdown structure will be necessary to enable you to make an estimate of how long each activity will take. You might need to make some inquiries before you can make a reasonably accurate estimate if the work requires delivery of materials or time to complete specialist processes. It is worth spending time in trying to make the estimate as accurate as possible at this stage, because the scheduling plans will be based on this information. Although it is almost inevitable that you will have to make changes as events unfold, it is annoying to have to do this when a little more work at an earlier stage could have provided a more realistic foundation.

**Example 8.2 – Time estimates for relocation of an office**

This example shows the time estimates for the activities identified in Example 8.1.

| **Activities** | **Estimated time in weeks** |
|---|---|
| **1. Prepare the site** | |
| 1.1 survey site | 1.1 about 3 weeks (needs discussions and an expert) |

| | | | |
|---|---|---|---|
| 1.2 | plan alterations | 1.2 | only 1 week once we have the information |
| 1.3 | estimate building work | 1.3 | 1 week because we'll need to call builders in |
| 1.4 | contract builders | 1.4 | 2 weeks because we need three estimates and decision |
| 1.5 | purchase building materials | 1.5 | 1 week because builders will normally do most of this |
| 1.6 | carry out building work | 1.6 | about 4 weeks to knock down walls and partition |

**2. Furnish and equip office**

| | | | |
|---|---|---|---|
| 2.1 | plan furnishing needs | 2.1 | 2 weeks because it needs discussion with staff |
| 2.2 | identify what we have | 2.2 | 2 weeks – could be done in same discussions |
| 2.3 | purchase furniture | 2.3 | this normally takes 3 weeks to deliver |
| 2.4 | plan equipment needs | 2.4 | 2 weeks – similar discussions with staff needed |
| 2.5 | identify what we have | 2.5 | same 2 weeks |
| 2.6 | purchase equipment | 2.6 | allow 3 weeks |
| 2.7 | install furniture | 2.7 | time to pack, move and re-site 1 week |
| 2.8 | install equipment and connect | 2.8 | allow 1 week as we'll need to test it all |

**3. Service preparation**

| | | | |
|---|---|---|---|
| 3.1 | plan service during the move | 3.1 | 2 weeks, needs discussion to share space |
| 3.2 | inform service users | 3.2 | 2 weeks, need to discuss who and tell them |
| 3.3 | arrange resources needed | 3.3 | 2 weeks, might do this in same discussions |
| 3.4 | deliver service during move | 3.4 | 1 week duration of move |
| 3.5 | prepare new staff locations and rotas | 3.5 | 2 weeks, could be tricky and a lot to arrange |
| 3.6 | prepare info about new location | 3.6 | 3 weeks because we'll need to print new stationery |
| 3.7 | inform when move completed | 3.7 | 1 week as this can all be done by e-mail and letter |

As some of these activities had a lot of separate tasks, the project manager checked each of these estimates against the task list to ensure that everything had been considered.

The level of detail in planning the schedule depends, as always, on the level of complexity of the project. People who are used to organising changes might look at these planning lists with horror, thinking that much of this is 'common sense' and that it makes things look more complicated than they are. Another point of view is that if one person carries all of this detail in their head, it is very difficult for anyone else to understand what is happening or to do anything helpful in their absence. The planning approaches can be chosen to accommodate the way in which the sponsor wants the project to be carried out. If wide support and collaboration are required, it is usually important to share information widely and to involve others in making decisions that will affect them.

Once the times have been estimated for each activity, it is possible to draw up a detailed schedule. You will probably have made a Gantt chart by this time and you may like to revise it in the light of the information that is now available. The revised Gantt chart may give enough information for you to go ahead without any further scheduling if timing in the project is not a particular concern.

If the time-scale is important, there is a technique that can help you to be much more precise about the timing of each element and the sequence in which they need to be completed in order to complete the whole project in the shortest possible time. This is called 'critical path analysis' and is sometimes referred to as CPA. The critical path is the shortest possible time in which the project can be completed once the timing of each task and the necessary sequencing has been taken into account. The activities and their timings can be drawn onto a chart that shows the paths that each activity must take and their relationships to each other. In particular, this chart shows the dependencies, that is when one activity cannot start until another is completed. It is

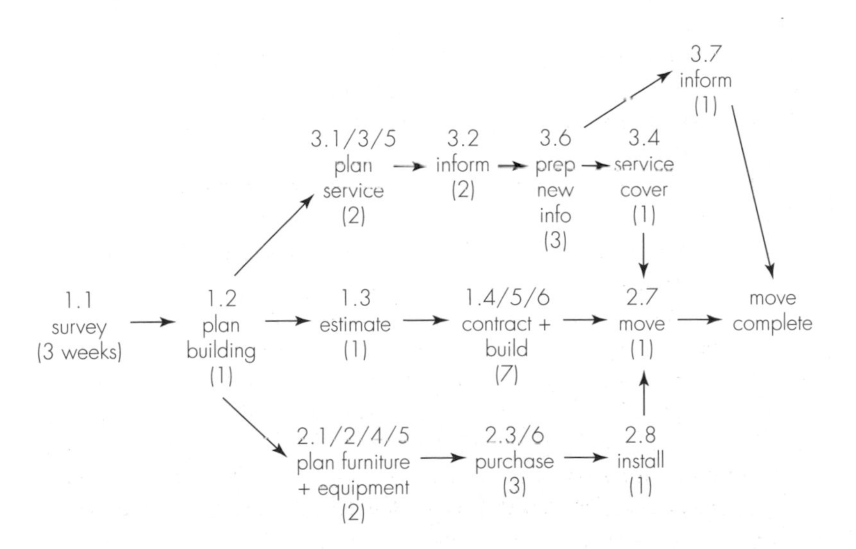


Figure 8.2 Critical path for relocation of an office

usually the impact of dependencies that slows a project down, so the dependencies and the resulting sequence need to be identified in order to establish the critical path.

You may need to draw out the diagram several times before you can show the sequence clearly. The sequence of activities in package 1 (prepare the site) is the easiest one to draw first because each activity is dependent on the previous one. For example:

- 1.1 (survey the site) has to come first;
- 1.2 (plan alterations) cannot happen until the survey information is available and any necessary decisions about building work to be carried out are made;
- estimates of the costs of building work (1.3) cannot be made until the plans are complete and specifications produced;
- three estimates must be obtained and a decision made about which builder should be awarded the contract before the contract can be agreed (1.4);
- 1.5 (purchase building materials) cannot be completed until the contract is signed because this is usually done by the builders according to the specification;
- all of this has to be completed before building work can commence (1.6);

and this sequence has to be completed before the office move can happen.

Package 2 (furnish and equip the office) cannot start until the alterations have been planned because these will determine the space in which furniture and equipment will have to fit. Staff will want to understand the opportunities and restrictions of the new office space before they can comment on the furnishing and equipment needs in any detail. It is also safer to wait until the alteration plans are complete before starting on package 3 (service preparation) because any staff involved will find it difficult to discuss changes in working practices until they have some idea about the length of time that the service will be disrupted.

A number of activities in packages 2 and 3 can be completed while the building work is in progress, but some cannot be progressed until the new office is ready for occupation. At that stage, the furniture can be installed (2.7) whether it has been moved from the previous location or has been purchased as new. Similarly, the equipment can be installed (2.8) once the electric wiring has been completed, although some equipment may need furniture to be in place first. During the week of the move the normal office service will be covered by a temporary service (3.4) which has to be arranged and resourced in time for that period.

The service cannot be provided from the new office until all of the activities have been completed. This diagram shows the sequence in which that has to happen and the length of time each activity will take.

To find the critical path, you look for the stages in the sequence where something must be completed before others can progress. In this diagram 1.1 (surveying the site) must start first and be followed by 1.2. Once 1.2 (planning the alterations) is complete, a number of other activities can start. These include 1.3, 2.1, 2.2, 2.4, 2.5 and 3.1. These activities all have paths that lead to completion of the building work, but each path takes a particular length of time to arrive at that stage. The activities in package 1 take the longest in total, with 1.3, 1.4, 1.5 and 1.6 taking eight weeks in total. The next longest take up to five weeks, so there is some choice about when these are carried out during that overall eight-week period. Activity 3.5 (prepare staff locations and rotas) is a little different because that will not be needed until the new office is ready for staff to begin to deliver the service from there, although these matters are usually agreed well in advance because they can arouse strong feelings. A crucial stage is reached when the building work is complete because the furniture (2.7) and the equipment (2.8) can be installed. During this week the temporary service (3.4) must be provided and everyone who needs to know about the new office location can be informed (3.7). The critical path is the line that takes longest to reach each point at which further activities are dependent. The line in this project is 1.1, 1.2, 1.3, 1.4, 1.5, 1.6, then one week during which four activities take place. This critical path adds up to thirteen weeks, by the end of which time the office can be occupied and used.

It is important to have some idea of the length of time the project will take in the early stages of planning if the time of completion is critical. In a project of this nature, it is possible to reduce the critical path a little by investing more resources. For example, the length of time the building work will take might be reduced if more staff were engaged in the work, but it is not usually possible to speed up the drying time of plaster. The installation of furniture and equipment might also be completed more quickly if necessary, but may need more resourcing and possibly the services of an external contractor. As you can see, the balance of time, cost and quality is always an issue in considering project planning.

If you do make changes to the schedule to reduce the length of time one or more of the activities takes, be careful to consider the impact this has on the critical path. For example, in this diagram it would not create any advantage to carry out an activity more quickly if it was not one of those on the critical path. However, if enough time in the activities on the critical path was to be reduced, the path itself might change. In this example, if the current critical path was to be reduced to take less than ten weeks, the path of 1.1, 1.2, 3.1 and 3.5 might become the critical path, but there are also two other paths that would take ten weeks (the paths to install furniture and equipment). All of the estimated times on these paths would have to be considered in order to establish whether any other time could be reduced so that the shortest possible critical path time could be identified.

Although it is essential to identify dependencies, it is very helpful to establish those that are unavoidable. If one activity is usually completed before another it is not necessarily essential to complete it first and it might be possible to overlap the activities. It is an advantage to reduce the number of dependencies because that will increase the flexibility available in implementing the project.

A project manager does not always have a personal choice about what approach to take because of the number of other people who are involved in a project. There is no reason, however, why you should not make your own choice to work things out for yourself before you produce information in the form required by others.

These examples illustrate the use of this technique in a fairly simple way and hand-drawn diagrams would suffice to support planning. In more complex projects it is usual now to use computer software that helps you to draw these diagrams and enables the detail of tasks to be included with the activities. The greatest advantage with computer programmes is the opportunity to try out the impact of making changes much more quickly than would be possible if each new diagram had to be hand-drawn. However, the time needed to learn to use new software is a consideration for someone who may not often have to manage complex projects. There is also an issue of understanding and some people find that puzzling out a hand-drawn diagram helps them to think all of the issues through in a way that does not necessarily happen when feeding the information into a computer.

## ACTIVITY 8.1

*Allow 5 minutes.*

Check your understanding. If a task on the critical path is expected to finish five days early, will the project complete five days early?

Tick box ❒ Yes ❒ No

The answer is no, because there might be another task that was not critical in the original planning because it would have finished two days before this unexpectedly early one. In this case, this other task now becomes the critical one and defines the expected finishing time which would now be three days early.

CHAPTER 9

# IMPLEMENTING THE PROJECT

Implementation is an exciting time for people managing projects. It is the point at which all the planning begins to turn into practical outcomes. The nature of the work of a project manager changes at this stage from imagining how things will work into supporting the activities. The focus of attention moves from developing frameworks to monitoring the real activities to ensure that everything is progressing as planned. The attention of those managing projects can never stray far from planning because this is the mechanism by which we are able to keep the balance between time, cost and quality. Even when implementation is about to start, there is a little more planning to complete to ensure that the transition from planning to activity is smooth and effective.

## DRAWING UP THE IMPLEMENTATION PLAN

The implementation plan consists mainly of the plans that have already been completed. You will need to monitor progress against these plans and to take action to revise the plans as events interrupt progress towards achieving the project's objectives. The plans you should have at this stage are:

- the project brief with agreement about the goals and objectives of the project;
- a list of the deliverables;
- agreement about how the project will be managed, reported and reviewed;
- the estimates and budget;
- details of the people who will work on the project;
- details of the accommodation, equipment and materials available;
- the schedules, probably described in logic diagrams, Gantt charts and critical path;
- the risk and contingency plans.

You may not yet have an evaluation plan, although you should be clear about how success will be measured. The evaluation plan can be considered at review meetings. It is useful to think about it before the project progresses too far because you may want to collect data about performance and any problems encountered as you go along rather than trying to remember these things much later.

To move from planning into action you will need to plan how action will be taken and by whom. You will have to ensure that each task starts on time and that the necessary resources are available when needed. The day-to-day routines of the project will have to be managed and monitoring will take place throughout the implementation phase. A number of techniques can help managers of projects to monitor progress and to control projects so that the balance of time, cost and quality is maintained. As no two projects are alike, different approaches are necessary in different circumstances.

## TEAM STRUCTURE

Teams have great difficulty in working effectively if they are too large for their members to work together conveniently. Six to eight people is often considered to be about right. If the project needs more staff in order to deliver all of the outcomes, the structure could consist of a number of teams, each with a team leader. The team leaders would also form a team themselves to co-ordinate the project. In some projects there may not be a team but, instead, a number of individuals or groups making specialist contributions at an appropriate time. In either case, the task of co-ordinating inputs is vital.

It is not necessary to name all of the team members when structuring the staffing for the project. It can be helpful to identify people in terms of the expertise or skills that are needed to complete each of the main tasks. If there is a need to recruit members to the team, this process will help to identify the criteria for selection. If some of the project team have already been identified, or if the team leaders have been appointed, there is an opportunity to include them in determining the team structure. At this stage, the key responsibilities can be allocated.

If the project is complex, several people will need to hold responsibility for supervising activities. Once the team structure has been agreed it should be easier to decide who holds the different levels of authority. These will include identifying who holds authority to approve release of resources and completed work, who must be consulted about what and who must be informed. In some projects it might be appropriate to allocate authority for recording and storing information or for ensuring security.

The project manager will usually retain overall responsibility for ensuring that the plans are carried out. Once the levels of authority have been decided, it is not difficult to decide how the approval will be sought and recorded, how those who should be informed will be told and how consultation will be arranged. All of these activities involve sub-tasks that can be allocated to individual team members.

## PLANNING TEAM RESPONSIBILITIES

It is important to give clear allocation of roles and responsibility for each task and key stage. This ensures that each piece of work is 'owned' by a particular person who will be accountable for completing it or seeking help if a problem develops. Planning these responsibilities also helps to ensure that overall responsibility for the work is spread appropriately between members of the team.

It is also important to establish clear lines of accountability for each team member. The arrangements will vary according to the size and complexity of the project, but each person needs to know:

- what is expected of them, possibly written as objectives with time-scales;
- the extent of the authority they have to make decisions about their area of work;
- the person who will act as their line manager for the duration of the project;
- the arrangements and frequency for reporting and reviewing progress.

If the project is large enough to have team leaders for different activities, it is important to check that each of these understands how the work of their team fits into the overall plan. It can be helpful to give each team leader their section of the plan detailing what should be achieved by specific dates. The milestones identified earlier in the plans will provide a useful check-list of outcomes and the dates by which each should be completed.

## MAKING IT HAPPEN

It is often quite difficult to start work on a project. The focus changes from planning to action. Even when tasks are allocated and the scheduling is complete, staff will not automatically start working on the tasks. It is usually up to the project manager as the leader of the project to ensure that work starts. It is important to make sure that everyone knows who should carry out what tasks and when each should start. The staff must be free to begin work and the essential materials and equipment need to be available. Even then, it is often necessary to support staff to start the work.

It can be helpful to start with a meeting to ensure that everyone understands the plan and where their contribution fits into the whole project. Planning is often focused on time-scales and schedules and team members may not be able to interpret the plans to find out exactly what they should be doing. This is particularly true when plans have been computer-generated and look daunting to people who are not used to working with them.

**Example 9.1 – Understanding the plan**

A senior nurse had decided to hold a workshop to begin the project because the team had not met and she thought it was important to develop a shared understanding of how the project was intended to progress. After the meeting she commented, 'I had made a huge assumption and had to change how I ran the workshop. I thought that they all knew about our organisational structure and strategy. There has been so much information given out recently about the new strategic direction. However, once I started making the introductory presentation I could see from their blank faces that they didn't have a clue what I was talking about. I had to change the workshop plans completely and start from much further back than I'd intended. I had to explain how the organisation worked and where we were going before they could begin to understand what the project was about or why it mattered.'

Once you are sure that everyone has sufficient understanding of the plans, you can start work. The key people responsible for carrying out each task need to know exactly what is wanted and you may have to confirm this with each individual. In some settings it will be necessary to ensure that all the formalities have been completed to secure the involvement of the team members. It may sometimes be necessary to issue a formal instruction before people are able to start work.

## RESOURCING

Even when all the necessary physical resourcing has been agreed and planned with an adequate budget, it will often fall to a project manager to take care of practical details and to encourage everyone to take action. There are times when it is worth doing something yourself to demonstrate support and commitment and to provide the means for others to start work.

Work will be impeded or interrupted if the necessary materials and equipment are not readily available or if the accommodation for the project has not been arranged. The project manager is usually responsible for resource allocation and utilisation, but if resources can be clearly linked to areas of responsibility, the relevant budgets can be delegated. By conferring responsibility to achieve an outcome within the budget a direct link between costs and outcomes is established.

Some resources have to be managed by qualified people. For example, if the project requires the handling of specialist equipment or the use of restricted drugs there are statutory requirements to observe. In setting up the project responsibilities it may be necessary to identify people with particular qualifications or experience to manage specialist areas of work.

## MANAGING PROJECT ACTIVITIES DURING IMPLEMENTATION

The main activities that the project manager has to consider during implementation are:

- managing communications and information;
- reviewing progress through monitoring and reviewing progress against the plan;
- controlling progress – using the information developed through monitoring and reviewing to decide when action needs to be taken to either bring the progress of activities closer to the plan or to change the plan;
- taking action in whatever way is appropriate when it is necessary;
- managing change, both the changes resulting from carrying out the project in its environment and the changes made to the project activities or plans during implementation.

The key information to communicate as implementation begins is the element of the plan that will be completed by each individual and team. Even if people have been involved in the development of the plans, you cannot assume that they understand the whole picture or even the part of it that is their responsibility. Many project managers take particular care to ensure that staff understand what they are expected to do, the standards expected and the length of time the activities should take. There is also an opportunity in this early stage to set up communication channels and to demonstrate the style in which you expect communication to be carried out during the implementation activities.

Much of the work of the project manager focuses on monitoring and control. Monitoring is the regular collection of information about the progress of activities. The information collected has to be compared with the planned progress so that any difference can be identified. If work is falling behind schedule, it may be necessary to take action to bring the project back into control. This is a crucial set of activities during implementation because it is the only way that a project manager can be sure that the project will finish successfully on time, within the budget and achieving all of the objectives intended.

There will certainly be change during the implementation stage of the project. All of the project activities are in themselves planned to cause a change. These are often complex and difficult to manage, but careful planning, monitoring and control will help you to manage these aspects effectively. Leadership, team-working and performance management also contribute to keeping the implementation stage moving forward in a positive and productive way.

There can also be change in the immediate environment of a project that impacts on the activities or objectives of the project. In some cases, external change can be predicted and will have been thought about when compiling the risk register. If this is the case, there will be some guidance about what action to take. If the change was not anticipated and appears of particular significance, a project manager would normally seek the advice of the sponsor or a senior manager before taking any action that might alter the direction or balance of the project.

## KEEPING AN OVERVIEW

The position of a project manager is privileged in that he or she has access to every aspect of the project. In some ways, this means that it can be a lonely role. Although issues can be discussed with those concerned, people are not always prepared to share concerns widely, particularly if they feel embarrassed. A project manager will usually be trusted with a lot of confidences. Confidentiality is essential, both in formal management of information and in management of 'softer' information. When people are working informally it is not unusual to be drawn into situations in which one group are discussing another and if the project manager is seen to be 'taking sides' it will be difficult to maintain a position of trust. Most project managers, even very experienced ones, need support sometimes from someone who can take a more distant perspective. It can be very helpful to have a mentor with whom to discuss things in confidence.

**Example 9.2 – Managing 'soft' information**

A manager reflecting on a project he had managed commented that one of the difficulties had been poor documentation of information that had not seemed very important at the time it was collected. He had gathered a great deal of information in the early stages of the project through discussion with staff, who occupied many different roles from front-line service delivery to senior management. He had even interviewed directors and the Chief Executive. Sometimes he had also gained valuable insights from chance informal meetings in corridors. He also realised that much of his information had been derived from observation as he had spent considerable amounts of time in the work areas that were to be affected by the project. Unfortunately, he had only made notes in the more formal interview situations and these were always of rather specific things that people had said. Much of his real information had come from how they had said it or from the hopes and fears that were expressed. He had not made notes from the observations at all, nor of the sudden insights that had been prompted informally.

He commented that, seen retrospectively, much of this was very useful information and would have helped the implementation stage although it had been collected with the planning in mind. He had not realised the value of this information throughout the project and wished that he had recorded it in some way that would have enabled him to retrieve it at later stages. As much of it had been rather 'soft' and probably very much influenced by his own perspectives, he commented that he wished he had kept a personal journal or file, so that he could remind himself of the ideas that had emerged. This would have been particularly useful when he was writing the final report and wanted to identify what had been learnt from the project.

This range of responsibilities can seem quite overwhelming for a person managing a project for the first time or even for someone with some experience. It is usually the role of the project manager to initiate all of these activities and to ensure that they happen, but they do not all have to be carried out by one person. It is usual to carry out reviews with the involvement of key people, so different perspectives can be taken into consideration. These people will also often be the ones who can carry out amendments once the group has decided that action should be taken. The project manager's main concern during implementation is to keep an overview of the whole project and to ensure that the balance of time, cost and quality is maintained while the activities of the project progress towards a successful conclusion.

CHAPTER 10

# MONITORING AND CONTROL

In an ideal world, projects would be completed on time, within specified budgets and to the standards set out in the plans. In practice, any project involves a set of unique problems and constraints that inevitably create complexity and risk. Plans are liable to change as work progresses and each stage in the process may have to be revisited several times before completion. Although projects have boundaries that protect them to some extent from other activities in the environment, external events will affect the project. The rapidly changing environment of health and social care may have significant impact on longer projects and may require not only revision of project plans but also some realignment of objectives. In any project, new issues will emerge as activities evolve. It falls to those leading and managing projects to be aware of events that impact on the project plan (*monitoring*) and to revise the plans if necessary (*controlling*).

There are a number of ways of monitoring a project during its progress to identify any emerging risks or potential for improvement. Monitoring is essential to collect appropriate information to inform the project manager about anything that threatens to disrupt the project and to stop it from progressing according to the plan. Once the project manager knows that there is a problem, a decision can be taken about how to address the problem. Action can be taken to ensure that activities are kept in line with the plan or the plan can be changed. Taking action to control the project ensures that the focus is kept on achieving the outcomes within the budget and time-scale agreed.

Some people in health and care services are nervous about the idea of controlling performance. The word 'control' sounds very authoritarian and inflexible. However, control in projects is essential if outcomes of the right quality are to be achieved within the time and budget agreed. All projects need investment of resources to take place at all and in health and social care services staff are well aware of the need to make good use of scarce resources. Control is part of effective management and is a key responsibility of a project manager.

# MONITORING

It is not 'cheating' to change the plan, because the environment is always changing and new information becomes available as a project progresses.

To control a project you need a plan that details how things should be happening and you need accurate information about what is actually happening. Monitoring is the activity of collecting information about the progress of activities and comparing this information with the plan to identify any differences. Once these variations have been identified, the project manager can consider whether there is any cause for concern. In some cases, the variations will be within the tolerance that the plan allowed and there will be no need to take action. If the progress of activities is very different from the plan, you will need to take action. Action should be taken when there is a danger that the project will not meet its targets because progress is too slow or if a delay in one activity will impact on others causing waste and further delay. Control may be regained either by taking action to change the progress of the activities that vary from the plan or by revising the plan to accommodate the variation in the progress of activities.

Control is about monitoring progress and taking timely corrective action. However sound your project plan, it is certain to need adjusting and updating as you go along. There are techniques that help to make this possible.

The process of project control is a simple loop (see Figure 10.1). The four stages in this loop are:

1 The project plan. The plan is a dynamic collection of documents that show the current plan and also record successive changes in the plan.
2 Monitoring. This is the process of collecting appropriate information about the progress of the project and the setting in which the project is evolving.

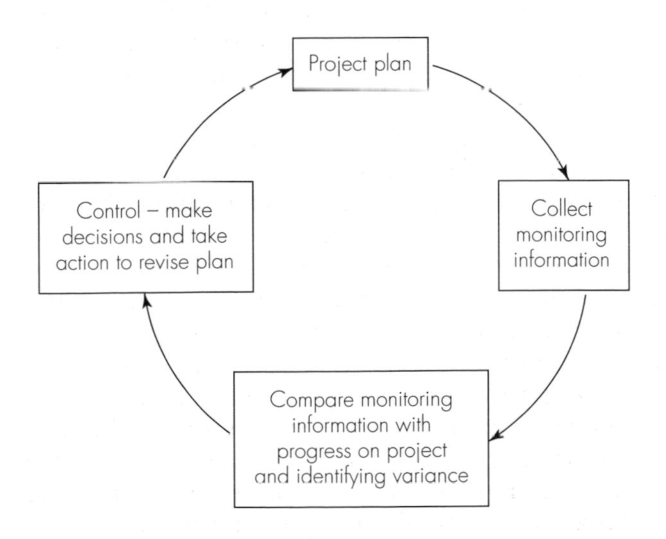


Figure 10.1 Simple project control loop

3 Identification of variance. This is the process of comparing what is happening with the plan to identify any variation from the plan.
4 Control. Decisions are made about how to address any variance. The risk register may already have identified potential responses. If this has not already been discussed, authority may have to be obtained before action can be taken. The two usual options are to invest more resources than were originally planned to enable tasks to be completed more quickly or to extend the time-scale to accommodate slower results than were planned. In either case the plan is changed and changes have to be recorded.

Expect change. Expect that as the project progresses there will be things that you will want to change within the boundaries of the project. There will also be changes in the environment of the project that will impact on the tasks and activities that are part of the project itself. Whenever a review of the project progress leads to a decision to make a change in the plan, it is essential to record the changes on the plan itself so that a master plan is maintained that is up to date. If you don't do this, you will be measuring progress against the original intention rather than against the revised plan and there is great potential for confusion. If you always record changes to the plan you will maintain a 'living' document as the basis for continuing action.

Successful control of a project depends on the flow of information, so it is important to have systems in place to make sure that you get feedback on what is happening. However, monitoring is not a solitary activity carried out by the project manager. If the project team meets regularly to review progress, monitoring becomes more dynamic and changes to the plan can be achieved by consensus. Involving the team not only helps to keep everyone on target – it also builds commitment.

Monitoring is the most important activity during the implementation phase of a project because it is the only way in which you can control the work to be sure that the objectives of the project will be met. To keep track of what is happening you may have to consider gathering information on two levels:

- 'Big picture' level – to include overall business objectives to which the project is intended to contribute and the balance of the dimensions of time, budget, quality;
- 'Project activity' level – to include tracking individual tasks: that they have been initiated, that they are running on track and that they are due to complete as planned.

In some ways it is quite difficult to pay attention to the 'big picture' issues when you are immersed in a project. It is easy to lose touch with what is happening in the rest of the organisation, particularly when constant change means that people have little time to think of anything other than the immediate pressures of work. It is important to stay alert to the broad direction of change in your service or organisation, because any projects within the setting should be helping to move in the right direction and not doing something that once seemed important but is no longer needed. It would be unusual for a project to be so out of date that it was found to be completely redundant, but it is possible that some of the objectives were agreed before new information caused a slight change of direction.

You will probably have to use a variety of means to gather the information you need to track the progress of the project. Project status reports and project status meetings are formal reporting structures that enable you to collect and collate this information. However, if you rely on others to provide all of your information you may miss early signs of difficulties – many experienced project managers make a point of 'walking the project' to keep in touch with the day-to-day realities that emerge as work progresses.

---

## ACTIVITY 9.1

*Allow 5 minutes.*

What might you be able to monitor as a project manager by 'walking the project' that you would not know about from formal reports?

________________________________________

________________________________________

________________________________________

________________________________________

________________________________________

By keeping a level of informal contact with the most important activities you will be better able to monitor the atmosphere in which teams are working. You will be in a better position to judge whether the interpersonal relationships are creating a productive energy or contributing to conflict and delay. You will be able to respond quickly if teams are facing delays because of failures in deliveries of materials or equipment. You will be more likely to notice if any staff are being pulled away from the project because of other work pressures.

---

Control is only possible if you have a plan against which to measure progress. If the plan is clear about what should be achieved and when, it is possible to monitor progress to be sure that each outcome is of the right quality and achieved at the right time.

# MILESTONES

The key stages of the project and the schedules should allow you to identify milestones. Milestones are measuring points used in reviewing the progress of a project. They are often descriptions of the extent of progress that should have been made by the review date. Sometimes the milestones might include deliverables or outcomes of activities that have to be completed early because others are dependent on them.

The project manager is often asked to set the milestones so that regular reviews can consider progress. It is, of course, wise to be cautious in proposing how much should have been completed by each review date. The first step in this case would be to decide when reviews should take place, perhaps monthly or quarterly, depending on the nature of the project. Then consult your plan to see what should have been achieved by each review date. These achievements can be listed for each review date as the milestones. The schedule will provide guidance, but it is often possible to allow a little more leeway in setting milestones so that some contingency is included. If you are setting milestones for the first time, look at the Gantt chart and the schedule and for each review date ask yourself what you want to see completed by then or how much progress you expect to have made. Milestones often include targets that are only part of a complete objective. For example, a milestone might set a target of 25 per cent of registrations completed for a training course when the full target is not to be achieved until two months later.

Milestones can be set in different ways, to reflect slightly different purposes. Milestones are often used to provide an agenda for a regular meeting to ensure that the project is progressing satisfactorily. Some organisations take a more challenging approach and enquire at each review whether the project should be terminated, expecting an adequate defence to be made in terms of the continuing value of the project to the organisation.

Once milestones are established and agreed, they form the basis for discussions about the progress of the project. In a long project it is reassuring to be able to demonstrate progressive achievements through the milestones, especially if the outcomes of the project will not be visible until a much later date. Similarly, if any of the milestones are not achieved there is an opportunity to discuss the reasons and to revise the plan if necessary.

This systematic approach to project control provides a simple process of planning, measuring against the plan and taking action to bring things back into line if necessary. However, this suggests that events will move in a fairly linear way. Life is messier than this systems view would suggest, and every time that something happens it will have an impact on everything else around it – so it is also important to retain an overview.

## MAINTAINING BALANCE

A project manager is always concerned with balancing the costs, time and quality dimensions of a project. Monitoring provides the information that is necessary to understand problems that arise in any of these dimensions. Delay and poor time management are often a problem but this can have a direct impact on the costs of a project as well as on the quality of what is achieved within the time available. Because of the importance of these dimensions and the extent to which they affect each other, monitoring information is required about time spent on project tasks, the resources used in completion of each task and the extent to which quality standards are consistently achieved. Once monitoring has revealed that controlling action is necessary, there will usually be a number of options about what sort of action to take.

When time is likely to be a concern, you can plan so that any delay has as little impact as possible. For example, you might split the key stages to avoid one following another in sequence when there is no necessity to have one in place before the next. You can check whether the critical path requires the sequence or whether it was planned simply to reduce the need for more resources. If it is possible to carry out two or more key stages concurrently, you will speed the project up, but you will need to resource all of the concurrent stages rather than waiting for one to finish so that staff can be moved to the next stage.

If the budget is a problem, you might make savings by removing or reducing contingencies from estimates. As the project work progresses you could review the contingency time and budgets that you had originally estimated. You will be in a better position to judge how much contingency is likely to be needed as the project progresses in achieving milestones.

You could re-evaluate the dependencies in the schedule. You may have been too cautious in making the first judgements about the sequence of activities. As some outcomes are achieved, you may find that you can avoid some of the dependencies. You may also find that you can make more use of slack time to speed up completion of tasks. As the project develops you may find that you can minimise duplication to make savings of time and effort.

It may be necessary to renegotiate to increase the time-scales if an unanticipated problem has caused a delay that cannot be recovered. If this is considered, it is worth calculating whether increasing the time-scale would be more cost-effective than increasing the resources to enable completion on time. Increasing the resources available will usually increase the costs, so this should be considered alongside other options. It may be possible to increase resources with limited costs by reviewing the use of existing staff. For example, it may be possible to get new people with particular expertise assigned to a key stage that is falling behind schedule. However, you may already have these people within the team but carrying out activities that have less need of the expertise.

If a project is facing serious delays or is running over budgeted costs, it is worth considering the quality targets. It may be possible to reduce the quality or scope of specified outputs or outcomes. In considering this option, it is worth reviewing what quality means to each of the key stakeholders. It may be that additional features have been added to the project but that they will add very little value for the majority of stakeholders. In this case, it may be possible to add only the additional features where they will add value and not where they are irrelevant.

Monitoring of expenditure is another aspect of control. In many organisations the financial aspects of a project have to conform to the usual financial procedures of the organisation. There may be decisions to make about the number and levels of budgets and about how frequently budget holders should receive information about expenditure or report on their current position.

## CONTROLLING CHANGE

Sometimes a project sponsor will request an addition to the project that was not part of the original brief agreed. This can present a difficult situation for those who manage the project because you will want to maintain good relations with your client but you will also want to protect your budget and possibly a profit margin if you are a contractor for the work.

If your client requests a change, you need to assess the extent to which this will require additional time or resources. Specify the elements carefully and estimate the costs of carrying out the modification. It is possible that the change could be incorporated in the project plan within the existing time-scale and budget by adapting some of the tasks in the later stages of the plan. Once you are confident that you understand the implications of making the requested change in terms of time and cost, you can decide how to respond to the client.

You might decide to offer to make the change without any charge to the client. This depends to some extent on whether you are carrying out the project for a fee, to make a profit or not. You might decide that there is a case for making an additional charge and you will have the full costing for the modification to support your claim. You may want to negotiate with the client to achieve a solution that suits both of you, again with full understanding of the implications. If you are not working for a fee you may decide to make the change because it would add value without adding significantly to the costs. Whatever you decide to do, you will need to be fully informed of the cost and time implications of the proposed change before you enter discussions about how this will be managed.

Once any change has been agreed, review the project documentation. You may want to make a formal amendment to the project brief and you will have to amend the schedules and budgets and note changes in the plan. You will also have to communicate the changes to anyone who needs to take appropriate action.

CHAPTER 11

# COMMUNICATIONS

Effective communications are essential in maintaining progress and mutual understanding of issues that arise as the project unfolds. Many types of communication are necessary during a project, but it is always important to consider how to ensure that the flow of information works effectively. The reporting and review systems will provide a formal means of communication, but this is unlikely to be sufficient to meet all the needs of those working on the project or other stakeholders.

## COMMUNICATIONS IN A PROJECT

You may remember from the classic six-stage model of project management that communication is not a specific stage but provides a background for all of the project stages. Communication is necessary both to link each of the stages and within each stage. Communication is so central to the management of a project that poor communications can be considered a serious risk that would threaten the likelihood of completing the project successfully. For these reasons, it is important to consider how to manage the communications within a project.

One of the key concerns is the need to manage the information that has to be produced, collected and distributed as part of the project. The form in which information is recorded, stored and retrieved determines to a large extent how it can be used and by whom. The flow of information in a project needs to be planned to ensure that the appropriate information reaches the people who need it. The processes used to collect and distribute information will also have an influence on how well the information is communicated and understood.

The channels for communication in the project should include everyone who is involved. The project team will have to communicate with each other, as will teams completing different types of activities. There are also people outside the team who should be included, including the wider stakeholder groups and the sponsors.

Communication is a two-way process involving both giving and receiving. If we don't communicate with each other we may find ourselves working at cross-purposes. We would also lose the opportunity to influence and to be influenced by other ideas. For communication to work, the messages sent and received also have to be understood. There are many barriers to effective communication but if they are identified most of the pitfalls can be avoided.

Communication may be formal or informal, depending on the size of the project, the people involved and their usual ways of working, but it must happen if the project is to succeed. Team members can become immersed in their own activities and fail to seek or to listen to feedback from anyone outside the team. A comprehensive communications plan will consider how to provide mechanisms through which the essential two-way communication can take place.

Communication implies scope for some sort of dialogue, where messages are received, understood and given a response that might trigger a further response. Often the dialogue is to develop or to test understanding. If you send a message and are sure that it has reached its intended destination, you still cannot be sure that it has been given any attention or that it has been understood. Communications can be improved by:

- paying attention to the needs of other people;
- listening actively, taking care and noticing signs;
- taking time to communicate in an appropriate way;
- taking time to check that the message has been understood;
- paying attention to feedback;
- giving feedback;
- choosing the time and place when expecting to have a difficult or confidential conversation.

Communication is necessary to ensure mutual understanding. When you consider channels of communication in a project environment you need to consider how you, as the manager of the project, will receive and respond to messages as well as how you will send them out. This is particularly important in planning how information will be handled in the project, because you cannot be sure that the information you give is understood by the recipients until you hear the response or test out understanding in some way.

## WHY IS GOOD COMMUNICATION NEEDED?

The purpose of communication in a project is to explain to others what has been achieved and what remains to be completed and to listen and respond to the needs and views of others concerned with the project. The project manager is usually the person in the middle of the web of activities who is able to keep an overview and to ensure that communications flow openly through all the channels that are needed.

One of your main concerns as a project manager is to ensure that everyone who needs information receives the right information for the purpose at the time they need it. This can often be planned using each activity line on the schedule. Each person or team needs to know when they can start work and whether anything has arisen in the previous period of work that will affect the next period. This will often involve a mix of information including formal written plans and face-to-face meetings at important handover points.

Open and full communication with everyone involved in a project not only ensures that information is handled efficiently. Communication can be used to motivate by offering encouragement, praising success, reassuring when things are not going as smoothly as hoped and supporting those whose energy or confidence is waning. It can be powerful in engaging people to work enthusiastically towards achieving outcomes that they believe are worthwhile.

If the project involves interdisciplinary, inter-professional or inter-organisational working, the value of rich interaction cannot be overestimated. When people have very different experience, assumptions and backgrounds it is difficult to establish common ground so that there is enough trust and confidence in each other to work together effectively. Although face-to-face communication can reveal differences, there is also opportunity to identify similarities and shared concerns. If there is support for the purpose and aims of a project this can provide the opportunity to build shared understanding and to identify common ground in values and aspirations. If people develop enthusiasm to achieve a common goal it is much easier to work together.

## HOW CAN COMMUNICATION BE PROVIDED?

Project managers use a range of communication channels including face-to-face meetings, phone, written and electronic notes, presentations and reports. These different means of communication each have advantages and disadvantages and it would limit a project considerably if too few approaches were used.

**Example 11.1 – Day-to-day communication**

Jo was managing a project that involved several teams working in different locations. As she arrived at her office she found that one of the team leaders was waiting for her, wanting a brief chat before starting that day's work. She realised that she had to listen before he could get back to work, so focused on what he had to say. It concerned other staff, so she asked him into her office to maintain confidentiality. Once he had said what he had planned, he still seemed worried, so she arranged to meet him later in the day when they could both give a bit more time to the concerns.

This meant that she was ten minutes late when she was able to settle at her desk, but she had to make three phone calls before she did anything else. Her secretary had signalled that she needed a word and she alerted Jo to some other issues that were concerning staff on the project.

It was almost an hour later when Jo was able to look through her in-tray and found details of two items that had been referred to during the phone calls. She took several further phone calls while she checked what else was in the in-tray and opened her e-mail. Again, she found that there were several issues that recurred and it was helpful to read all the messages before she replied to any because they all concerned current issues.

Most project managers face this range of communications and need to spend time listening to the issues and noticing other signs of concern before making decisions or taking action. In most projects, what affects one area will have some impact on others. Sometimes these things run their course and are solved by those involved, but in other cases the manager of a project has to intervene to reduce the levels of anxiety or to solve a problem that is delaying work.

Much of the communication will probably be in the form of written words and charts and diagrams. This has the advantage of consistency in that everyone can be sent the same message. Unfortunately, this will not ensure that everyone receives the same message. We are all different and we all interpret messages differently. If a team is sent the appropriate part of a written project plan, there is no guarantee that they will understand it or the implications for their work. Moreover, they may feel neglected and unwelcome on the project if you don't meet them and go through the plans, listening to their concerns and offering personal support.

Formality and informality both have their place.

A formal message carries authority and may seem unnecessarily directive to someone who expects to be consulted and not 'told' what to do. Instructions can be issued in different ways and in some settings a face-to-face discussion and agreement can be much more effective than a string of threatening e-mail messages.

We send a lot of messages through our tone of voice, appearance and actions. Project managers who want their project to be successful will use all aspects of communication to support their aims. We are often not very aware of non-verbal communication, but it can be a strong influence on how people feel about the project. It is not as specific as use of words is intended to be, but people 'read' it in a very basic way that raises positive or negative and uneasy feelings. We can be aware of the reactions we are receiving from others and try to avoid misunderstandings before they damage the project. Openness about ideas and feelings is crucial to success in communities where a shared value base is important as in health and social care services.

## MANAGING THE FLOW OF INFORMATION

There are two main areas of information that need to be managed in a project. Plans are needed so that all those who need to know can be informed about what should happen, when and how. The other type of information is about what actually happens, so that completion of plans can be confirmed or revisions can be made. Those who are interested in the project or its outcomes will need both types of information. These people often include service users and the general public.

The key questions in planning the information flow are:

- Who needs information?
- What information do they need?
- Who can give it to them?
- When do they need it?
- Why do they need it?
- How do they need it?
- Where do they need it?
- What might hinder communications with them?

One way to identify the information needs is to work through the plans for each stage of the project considering who does what and what information is needed for them to do it. You can then consider how that information can be provided. To be useful, the information needs to be provided at the right time and in a format that is convenient.

## PROVIDING INFORMATION FOR THOSE WHO NEED IT

In the defining stage of a project the emphasis is on developing understanding through many different types of communication. The purpose of the project has to be clarified and agreed by the sponsors and key stakeholders. There may be a need for wide consultation if the project is likely to have implications for different groups of people.

Consultation cannot take place unless some basic information is supplied, even if this is in the form of a broad proposal and some options to consider. As feedback is received, the ideas can be refined and options both deleted and added. The information that is developing about the project has to be defined in a process similar to the process of defining the project itself. For the purposes of managing the project this information is recorded in the form of plans, but when information is to be shared it has to be prepared in a form that can be understood by those for whom it is intended.

Whether the project is small or large and complex, the information used in it needs to be of a high quality. Good information is:

- relevant (it is the information needed for the purpose);
- clear (presented in clear language and format);
- accurate (without mistakes and not misleading);
- complete (as much as is needed with nothing missing);
- timely (up-to-date information sent and received at an appropriate and helpful time);
- appropriate (the right information sent and received by the right people).

Remember, however, that sending out information is only part of the communication process and that many who receive information will respond and react in some way. Be prepared to interact with anyone to whom you send information.

**Example 11.2 – Effective meetings**

Effective communication involves giving information, collecting information and listening to people. To ensure the smooth running of your project, you might need any or all of the following:

- formal minuted meetings that run to a schedule appropriate to the project;
- meetings with your sponsor (which might be on a one-to-one basis);
- progress meetings with the project team or teams;
- individual meetings on a one-to-one basis with team members;
- problem-solving meetings arranged when particular issues need to be resolved.

Meetings need a clear purpose and focus and the formal ones should be recorded on project schedules. They should be time-limited and given proper priority in diaries so that time is not wasted waiting for inputs from key people. Meetings will be respected only if they are managed to avoid waste of time and effort.

Your stakeholders will expect to receive reports at regular intervals, whether formally or informally. So you need to ask yourself:

- Who needs to be informed?
- About what?
- How often?
- By what means?

> Meetings will not always be the best means for conveying information, but they will almost certainly be needed from time to time to ensure that there is shared understanding of any issues that arise during the progress of the project.

During implementation, information is needed continuously to monitor and control the progress of the project. Formal reports about the project status are often used to inform the monitoring process. Formal reviews are often held so that an overview of progress is regularly considered. Most projects need some system of reporting that provides regular and up-to-date information about what tasks have been completed and any problems that have arisen. These are often called project status reports.

## PROJECT STATUS REPORTS

Project status reports are regular formal reports. You can decide how often these are necessary depending on the size and nature of the project, but they are usually weekly, monthly or quarterly. Reports may even be required hourly if a problem is causing serious concern and has the potential to seriously delay progress. Daily reports might be necessary if there are implications for arranging work for the following day. Consider the degree of risk involved as a guide for deciding the frequency of reporting. The key issue is how quickly the project could get out of control and the time it would take to implement contingency plans. Also, the project sponsor might have a preference about the frequency of reports and review meetings.

To write the report you will need information from members of the project team about completion of tasks and key stages and any delays or difficulties anticipated. If there will be a number of project status reports a standard report form is helpful. This might include:

- the project title;
- the key stage or task covered by the report;
- the name of the person responsible for this key stage or task;
- the date of the report;
- actual progress reported against planned progress towards project 'milestones';
- explanation of any delay or any remedial action taken;
- any anticipated concerns or any issues awaiting resolution;
- the milestones due in the next reporting period and the date of the next report.

Once you have set up a system for regular reporting you will probably have to make sure that it happens, at least in the early stages. Be prepared to chase up reports and to insist that they are necessary and must be presented on time.

In the closing stages of the project, information concerns completion of all the objectives and arrangements for handing over all the deliverables. The project activities have to be closed with all the appropriate documentation completed. Most projects have an evaluation in the closing stage or after completion and those carrying out the evaluation will often require information from all of the previous stages of the project.

Reporting often raises issues for those who receive the reports. You may want to consider that people often react with questions at the level of detail that you have offered. If you limit what you offer to target the key concerns from each perspective you are likely to reduce the extent to which you have to smooth anxiety or deal with misunderstandings!

**Example 11.3 – Overview and detail**

A junior estate manager who worked for a large training centre based in a hospital reported a personal experience of reporting at a different level. He said, 'I was asked to make a presentation to our Chief Executive about the relocation of our residential accommodation and I was very worried that he would ask me to explain why we were so far behind schedule. We had found asbestos in one of the ceilings and had immediately stopped work and called in specialists to remove it. This had, of course, delayed everything. In fact, all that the CEO wanted to know was whether we were going to keep to the revised schedule now. He was very pleased to hear that we had asked the specialists to check all of the other rooms that would be part of this move so that there would be no more nasty surprises. It made me realise that in reporting at that level I had to give an overview and show that we could stand back from problems and look ahead to make sure that we achieved the main outcomes as well as possible.'

If you are managing a project, you will be responsible for providing regular progress reports to stakeholders, whether as written reports or as oral reports and presentations at meetings. The information gained from internal project reports will be helpful in compiling reports, but you will probably want to present different types of reports to stakeholders with different types of concerns. For example, the project sponsor may be most concerned with the overall progress against goals, but stakeholders concerned with one group of project objectives may only want to see reports about that concern. Some stakeholders will have an interest only in the overview and the implications for their organisation.

## ACTIVITY 11.1

*Allow 10 minutes.*

What key questions do you think stakeholders would want you to answer when you prepare a report about the progress of the project?

1 ____________________

2 ____________________

3 ____________________

We think that the central questions are:

- Is the project on schedule?
- Is it within the allocated budget?
- Have the milestones been achieved?
- If not, what action has been taken to correct the situation?

Other questions may be appropriate, including ones about whether problems have been identified and solved, whether the experience so far has any implications for future plans, whether any additional resource is required or whether there is any need for revisions to the overall plan.

In many projects it is important to provide information not only to stakeholders but also to the general public. There is often interest in projects from external sources and information may have to be provided to the news media and to public interest bodies. Again, you can ask yourself what they will want to know. There is likely to be more interest in whether the project will present any sort of disruption or change and, if so, what the benefits will be.

In considering the timing of information releases, it is also important to consider what preparation is necessary to deal with reactions and responses. Large and powerful organisations can appear to be concealing planned changes if they do not offer information about plans until it is very obvious to everyone that changes are in progress. If it is possible, it is usually helpful to prepare information, perhaps in the form of press releases, to give to local community and media representatives. Sometimes a public meeting is appreciated so that anyone with concerns can raise them at an early stage.

Remember that the staff of any organisation involved in the project are likely to be the best ambassadors, but they may give out a very poor impression if they are not well informed and able to answer queries from those outside the organisation.

## WHERE IS INFORMATION NEEDED?

Information is often needed in locations remote from the project base. There is always a danger of focusing attention on staff information needs in the central base. If a project has staff and teams in other locations, it is important for face-to-face contact to take place sometimes and for the project manager to be seen in all the locations from time to time. Although telephone and e-mail are very convenient ways of sending and receiving messages, much richer communication is achieved when non-verbal interaction is also possible. One way of helping staff in remote locations to keep in touch is to rotate the regular review meetings from one location to another. If all staff are not included in the meeting, there could be a shared lunch with opportunities for social interaction.

The phases of the project present opportunities to hold celebratory events. These can be held in appropriate locations so that different aspects of the project are featured. For example, once your project plan has been prepared and agreed by your sponsors, there is an opportunity to launch the project with a celebratory event. Making the launch a special occasion provides the opportunity to bring the project team and other stakeholders together so that they can meet one another, perhaps for the first time, and form some informal networks that could facilitate the project. It is also an opportunity to establish your role as the project manager, and make sure everyone has a copy of the agreed, up-to-date project plan.

---

### ACTIVITY 11.2

*Allow 10 minutes.*

Make notes on how you would launch a project, including whom you would invite and what you would do on the day.

________________________________________

________________________________________

________________________________________

________________________________________

________________________________________

Every project launch is different, but you will need to arrange a suitable venue, considering how it will enhance the image of the project and ensuring that it is accessible for people with disabilities. You will have to send out invitations and this is an opportunity to demonstrate partnerships and collaboration by including appropriate names and logos. You will probably want the project's sponsor to open the meeting by setting the scene for the project, and explaining its priority and your role. On the day, you may have to:

- introduce people to each other;
- introduce the project team and their roles;
- explain the benefits of the project and its anticipated outputs and outcomes;
- describe the project plan;
- explain the procedures for communication;
- respond to questions.

Launching the project allows you to set the tone of communications during the event. You may arrange to be formal or informal, personally accessible or distant, friendly and open or closed and withdrawn. However you present yourself and the event sets the pattern for future communications.

## ACCESS TO INFORMATION AND CONFIDENTIALITY

If you are trying to establish a climate in which people communicate openly and share information readily, it is often difficult to manage information that should be kept confidential and only made available to those with authority to have access. It is helpful to consider in the early stages of a project what information must be kept confidential. If the project is within the context of an organisation or group of organisations, there may be policy guidelines that will govern management of information. If no guidelines are available to you, you must ensure that you observe the legal requirements. These change from time to time, but cover a number of areas that might be of concern in a project, including:

- the rights of individuals to see information held about themselves in personal files;
- only the data necessary for the purpose should be obtained and recorded;
- this data should be accurate, kept up to date and kept only for as long as is necessary for that purpose;
- the data should be used only for the purpose for which it was obtained.

If the project is taking place without the data management processes being under the umbrella of an organisation, the project may have to be registered to conform with the legal requirements. Personal data considered particularly sensitive include any information relating to racial or ethnic origin, political opinions, religious or other beliefs, trade union membership, health, sex life and criminal convictions. The legislation covers both paper and electronic records and if there is any doubt about whether the project activities conform to legal requirements further advice should be sought before any records are started.

Appropriate measures need to be taken to ensure that information is managed responsibly.

Once information has been gathered and stored it must be kept secure. The responsibilities include:

- Confidentiality. Access to data should be confined to those who need to know and have been given authority to view the data. If confidentiality is not maintained, the problem of disclosure arises and must be addressed.
- Integrity. Data must be accurate and complete if it is to be used effectively.
- Availability. Data must be available to be used when required by those authorised to use it.

The best defence to take against the risk of disclosure is to ensure that confidential records are kept securely and handled carefully so that access is always limited.

## WHAT MIGHT HINDER EFFECTIVE COMMUNICATIONS?

Barriers to communication exist in many forms. We all have favourite ways of communicating and ways that we are reluctant to use but may choose if they are likely to be more effective. Very common barriers to effective communications are:

- lack of clarity (in the message or in the way in which it is presented);
- poor transmission (for example, a phoned list of instructions when a written list would be better or written instructions when a demonstration would be better);
- failure to ensure that the message has been received and understood;
- failure to set up appropriate channels for communication (so people who should be in touch with each other don't know about each other's existence);
- misunderstanding (a message may be interpreted in a way different from that intended, sometimes as a result of being passed on several times);
- interference (a message has not been heard properly or attention was distracted because of noise, discomfort or distracting events);
- the person receiving the message didn't understand the importance of it because of their own background or circumstances.

Most of these barriers to effective communication can be overcome if care is taken to check that messages have been understood and that there is intention to take appropriate action. Remember that this works both ways and that you will often need to check that you have fully understood messages that you receive.

CHAPTER 12

# LEADERSHIP AND TEAMWORKING

It is difficult to define what makes a 'good' leader, but most of us would be able to distinguish between effective and weak leadership. Leading is associated with 'leading the way' and people who can see a way forward and are able to explain this to others and enthuse them to follow that path are often considered to be demonstrating leadership. In the language often used about leadership this translates as people who have vision and are able both to communicate the vision to others and to motivate others into taking action. Leadership is important in the initiatives intended to develop and improve health and social care services. This type of leadership is essential in projects.

Some people hold strong views about whether managers can or should be leaders and whether leaders can be effective without management skills. Many people are reluctant to propose that they might be a leader or lack confidence about whether they have the appropriate qualities and skills. There are style issues too, and the expectations in the context of a project will influence the selection of people for appropriate roles. The project manager is often also the leader in a project, but not always and not necessarily.

## THE NATURE OF LEADERSHIP

Leadership is essentially about relationships with other people. You can't be a leader unless others are prepared to go alongside you or to follow your lead. Traditional ideas about leadership have evolved through a range of different concerns. Early ideas about leadership associated leaders with heroism in battle and this has led to a view of leadership as single-minded, agressive, risk-taking and arrogant. These behaviours are not welcomed or appropriate in health and social care services that share basic values of respect for equality and social inclusion. Another traditional view that is equally unacceptable is of leaders being born with a natural ability into families that have powerful positions through generations of ownership of land and property.

More recent views have considered leadership as a role that is enacted in different ways in different contexts. It is widely acknowledged that there are different types of successful leaders. Many examples of different leadership styles prove successful when they are matched to particular circumstances. There has been a long-standing debate about whether leaders emerge naturally because it is a matter of personal characteristics, qualities and charisma or whether people can learn to be leaders. Increasing emphasis on the need for people able to successfully lead change in organisations has led to an expectation that managers, particularly senior managers, will be able to exhibit at least some of the characteristics of an effective leader. There is some consensus about what these characteristics are and they are usually described in terms of behaviour, competence or ability in relation to a particular context.

Different types of leadership are needed in different circumstances. This is not only a matter of personal style, but also reflects the nature of the setting and the direction of change. Leadership is often about leading day-to-day activities, but transformational leadership is valued when significant change is needed and both vision and direction have to be developed.

Leadership in a project is essentially about achieving aims within the boundaries of the project. A leader takes a particular role in the successful completion of a project, but this does not always have to be the project manager and in different circumstances different people might become effective leaders.

## LEADERSHIP IN A PROJECT

A project creates a context of its own because of its clear aims and boundaries that define what is inside the project and what is not. However, a project always exists in a wider environment in which events take place that can impact on the project and which the project can, itself, influence. Leadership in a project is about successfully achieving the intended outcomes agreed for the project. It might include successive revision of the nature of these outcomes if there is frequent relevant change in the wider environment. To achieve complete success, the activities of the project should respect the values of all those affected in any way. The focus is always on moving towards achievement of the project goals in a way that fully encompasses its purposes.

Leadership is essential in a project to develop the initial idea, gain support and funding, set the direction and strategy and to motivate and support the activities. All of these roles are also ones that a project manager often takes. A project provides an opportunity for people who would not normally take leadership roles in their day-to-day work to do so for the period of the project. For this reason, people are often asked to manage projects to gain experience in a leading role. A project manager does not, however, always have to lead every aspect of a project. It is often a senior person in a service or organisation who initiates a project and who frames the proposal in terms of purpose and key objectives and who secures support and funding before appointing a manager for the project. There may be experts in different fields who lead the activities that contribute to the project. There may be people who feel very strongly about the issues addressed by the project who lead in influencing stakeholders and shaping opinion about the value of the project. There may also be people who provide leadership in the teamworking necessary to co-ordinate the activities of the project. The manager of the project may take some or all of these roles.

A project can be successfully completed only if the people involved carry out all the necessary activities in a co-ordinated way. To achieve this, leadership and teamwork are necessary. Two aspects of leadership that affect the relationships between those in the various project teams are use of power and style of leadership.

# POWER IN LEADERSHIP OF PROJECTS

People with power can get things done and can stop things from happening. The use of power on groups of people can cause misery and fear or give the confidence of approval and protection. Leaders are often thought to be powerful people. Power is an energy that can be used in different ways according to the source from which the power is derived and the purposes and values of the person who holds the power. Power can be used to provide energy for your own activities or to empower others. You need some power to lead or manage a project because those who are to carry out the tasks and activities need to be empowered to do it. However, it is often more important to be able to work influentially within an environment where many people hold power than to hold substantial power yourself.

The source of power confers the power but also constrains its use. In a project there may be any of the following sources of power, each with related constraints. Individuals have several sources of power and the leader of a project is often concerned with how to access and co-ordinate the various contributions that others are empowered to make.

## Position power

The project manager has a title and role that confers some power but this is dependent on the extent to which the role carries authority to take decisions. The amount of authority held by project managers is crucial, as they will usually not be seen to hold enough power if they always have to ask permission of others before authorising expenditure or action. This is also true of team leaders and a project manager who holds considerable overall power can empower others through delegation of authority.

## Resource power

This is the power that derives from control of resources. Resources for a project may be agreed at a high level within an organisation, but it can still be very difficult for a project manager to access what is needed if those with power over the resources do not co-operate. For example, if staff are only part-time on the project and have line managers supervising their performance in other areas of work, the line managers have power over those staff as resources for the project. Such staff can feel that they are being treated as objects owned by others if they are caught in power struggles between project managers and line managers.

## Expert power

This is the power held by being an expert in an area of work. Many tasks and activities cannot be carried out without the skills, knowledge or experience of an expert. This can sometimes be a problem in a project if an expert seems inflexible and too bound by professional traditions in practice. In multi-professional teamworking there is often a need for leadership in negotiating between experts to enable appropriate actions to be taken to progress the project.

## Personal power

Everyone has the potential to influence others and the degree of personal power held is derived from the way in which others see you. Knowledge of yourself and the impact you make on others is very useful in understanding how much personal power you may have in different circumstances. It often takes time to establish personal power in a new situation or with new colleagues. Your self-confidence, sense of direction and enthusiasm influence others and are seen as leadership qualities.

## Information power

This derives from the information held by people and the extent to which they are prepared to share appropriate information with others. The power can, of course, be used to hold back information that would be useful if offered to others. One of the difficulties in managing a project is that relevant information will often be held in a number of different places and by different individuals. It can be difficult to identify the location of information as well as to gain access to it. Sometimes it is easier for other people to gain access because of their roles or areas of expertise. A project manager can often gain useful information by working with those who are willing and able to share.

### Political power

Some gain political power because they are elected to represent the views of others. Holding an elected position can carry considerable power whether the election is formal or not. For example, a community leader representing the views of a minority can become the leader of an influential pressure group. Informal political power can be gained by a person who is considered to have an ability to influence others. Power is not only 'given' but is often held because people allow it to be held by asking for suggestions or help or support from those who are perceived as able to offer it.

## STYLE IN LEADERSHIP OF PROJECTS

There is a fairly wide consensus that there is no one right way to be an effective leader. As every situation is different, leaders often have to be flexible about what style to adopt if they are to be able to balance the needs of the individuals, the teams and the task.

Style is often discussed as a continuum of possibilities between the opposing approaches of being very directive or consultative to the point of delegating decisions. A very directive style would be to tell everyone exactly what to do without discussing anything. The opposite would be a delegating style in which you hand over most, if not all, of the decision making. There are dangers in both of these extreme positions and most leaders and managers adopt a mixture of directive and consultative styles according to the situation and the people and tasks involved.

Some of the approaches that you can take come between a directive style and complete delegation. These include:

- selling – you explain your decision to staff and overcome any objections;
- shaping – you take the key decisions and then involve staff in shaping how to implement decisions;
- consulting – you invite comment and ideas and consider these in coming to key decisions;
- selective delegation – you delegate decisions within a framework that indicates the boundaries of the delegated authority. You also ensure that the person to whom you have delegated has the training and support to carry out the role.

In cultures where people are frightened of being blamed if mistakes are made it is important to ensure that individuals are not put at risk.

The further you come down this list of approaches, the more freedom you are perceived to be offering staff. Staff often prefer to have some freedom if they are well prepared for the responsibilities that involvement and delegation bring. It is important, however, to be aware of the expectations in any environment and to choose appropriate styles that will work for the people and objectives in the project. Delegation should be discussed and accepted by those to whom you want to delegate and support should be available to help them to succeed. Overall responsibility for achievement of the tasks that have been delegated has to remain with you.

## LEADERSHIP ROLES IN A PROJECT

Certain roles have to be taken by someone, often the project manager, in order to move smoothly through the phases of a project. The very important early stages involve developing the vision of the project in a way that encourages others to see its value. This vision has to be communicated to others and, once supported as a project, has to be turned into a set of plans that provide the strategy through which the objectives of the project will be achieved. The leader of a project then has to help everyone to maintain progress towards achieving successful outcomes – this is often likened to being a lighthouse and providing the beam of light that shows the direction and outcomes. The role of leader is often described as being concerned with vision and values and the role of the manager as ensuring effective and efficient actions. The role of the leader can be seen as to develop, communicate and maintain the vision, motivating everyone to progress in the right direction, while the manager ensures that the strategy is enacted with plans, activities and tasks that progress through a structured route to the desired outcomes.

Most projects, particularly those in health and social care settings, involve complex settings having many different views and expectations. In such settings it is always difficult to take action because people will be interested, concerned or vulnerable and there will usually be a need for negotiating skills.

**Example 12.1 Negotiating**

An experienced project manager made these comments about negotiating. 'There's no point in starting to negotiate unless both parties actually want to come out with a mutually acceptable agreement. That's the first thing to check. If someone tries to start negotiating but you are not prepared to concede anything or to envisage any changes, there is no room for negotiation. In a situation like that there is more work to do before you can move into a negotiating phase, if it is ever appropriate.

'Once you start to negotiate, you have to be ready to shift your position otherwise the other person will feel that all the movement is expected from them. It is important to be very clear about what is agreed and what concessions are made as you progress with discussions. There is usually a period during which you each make a few concessions, but you have to both feel that you are getting something in return. Negotiation only really works well if you are as concerned as the other person to ensure that you can both go back to your respective teams with something that they will recognise as a good outcome. That means respecting the other person and ensuring that no one loses face.

'That doesn't mean that we are always terribly nice to each other while we're in discussions. I've found that it is not unusual for people in negotiating meetings to use strong language and to lose their tempers on occasion. If you care a lot about something, that sort of behaviour is to be accepted and is usually tolerated.

'Whatever happens, I would always try to get to a conclusion that we are both pleased with and that can be written as an agreement so that everyone can progress with clear understanding and confidence that the terms of the agreement will be met.'

It is also the role of the leader to keep up enthusiasm for the project, particularly if there are long periods when nothing much seems to be happening even if all the milestones are being met. The evidence of progress against plans does not always shape people's feelings and perceptions. In health and social care services projects often seem to take energy away from the day-to-day work and this can be resented, particularly if there are no visible results. The role of maintaining the vision includes reiterating the value of the project and helping others to visualise the benefits it will bring. Some of the most successful leaders are those who are able not only to describe their vision to others but to help others see the vision for themselves in a way that enthuses them and energises them into action. Not everyone can be the sort of leader that can engage hearts and souls in a shared vision, but we can all contribute to motivation.

## MOTIVATION AND TEAMWORKING

It is ideal if all the staff on the project want to achieve the outcomes so much that they work enthusiastically and co-operatively towards those ends. Much has been written about motivation but there is general agreement that for people to be motivated, they have to feel that there will be some reward for their efforts. This reward need not be financial, in fact, that is usually not a particular consideration as long as the financial reward is fair for the conditions and range of work. It is often more important for people to feel that their work is worthwhile. In health and social care this is always important and people often talk about wanting to 'make a difference'. The rewards are in seeing that personal effort has contributed to improving another person's health or well-being.

The social interaction involved in collaboration to achieve worthwhile goals is often very rewarding in itself. Where there is opportunity for working together in teams, people are often motivated by having a productive role and sharing enthusiasm and support.

There are some things that leaders and managers of projects can do to maintain a high level of motivation in the project. In the early stages it is important to make sure that the purpose of the project is clear and that the contribution that everyone will make is explained. As things progress it is often useful to reiterate this, to ensure that everyone understands the value of the contribution made by each individual and team. It is helpful to develop ways of keeping everyone informed about completion of tasks and activities so that everyone can share in a sense of progress towards the objectives. Team members can be motivated by hearing about the successes that are achieved by others and can be rewarded by seeing reports of their own success shared widely within the organisation.

Although staff who work in health and social care services are usually very committed to the core values underpinning their work, these are not often discussed. It can be useful to encourage discussion of differences in values, perhaps between different professional or clinical groups, to discover where the common values bring people together. The values of the project should provide some common ground if everyone is committed to achieving them.

It can be productive and reduce discontent to encourage discussion of work practices and interaction both within teams and in wider interdisciplinary or inter-professional working groups. Differences can be significant if people have very different experience and professional or clinical training. If the teams are also multicultural, as is often the case, there may be many different views about effective ways of working. If there are difficulties, most people will be aware of them and either talking behind peoples' backs or trying to ignore problems. Neither of these behaviours are likely to be helpful in progressing the project, but regular discussions about shared practice can be constructive and illuminating.

## TEAM DEVELOPMENT

Building a project team is not a one-off activity that can be achieved through an 'away day', although this can be a useful mechanism. It is a continuing process that needs to be constantly worked at. The project team may be drawn from a variety of different departments within your organisation, or from different agencies, and may be very diverse in knowledge, skills and experience. Effective teamworking in a multidisciplinary context can be hindered by lack of understanding of each other's roles, but a project manager can ensure that there is opportunity and encouragement to explore the differences rather than leaving them partially recognised and potentially damaging to the project.

**Example 12.2 – Team building through developing the plan**

The creation of several Primary Care Trusts caused a Community Speech Therapy Department to consider how best to respond to the structural reconfiguration of services. The Head Speech Therapist considered that there were several opportunities for extending current services and arranged a half-day session for her staff with a facilitator to discuss the situation. The team all agreed that several opportunities did exist, but there was disagreement about where the opportunities lay. The Head Speech Therapist realised that these differences would not be resolved immediately. Two therapists felt that more research was required and the Head felt this was a good way to progress the decision-making process, recognising that such involvement would increase ownership and commitment to change.

The team developed a plan of action allocating responsibilities between them to seek further information to establish precise need. This involved arranging meetings with District Nurses, Health Visitors and General Practitioners from the Primary Care Trust. They also made visits to other Speech Therapy Departments operating in similar environments and met senior managers from the local Mental Health Trust (this was also identified as an expanding part of the health market). Finally the Head Speech Therapist and her Deputy agreed to design a questionnaire to survey existing and potential service users. The facilitator influenced the team members to set realistic time-scales for completion and a second session was arranged for three months' time. At the second meeting the team had gathered some important information, which ultimately focused their energies on planning the provision of new services in the community mental health setting.

(Stephen Oliver, Management Training Consultant,
Business Development Consultancy.)

Not all projects use teams to carry out the work, although we tend to talk about the project team. For some projects it is only necessary for individuals or groups to contribute a specific component after which there will be no further participation. This may happen when a project is concerned with very technical issues or when the area of work is very well understood and the project is not unusual. In most cases, the context of health and social care services is so complicated that people working on a project have to collaborate in order to achieve anything.

Some of the most important characteristics of a successful team are:

- working together to achieve a common goal;
- caring about the contributions made by others;
- awareness that more can be achieved through collaboration than through individual effort;
- sharing of vision and values that maintain motivation.

It is not easy to achieve all of these.

Teams take some time to develop and have to progress through formative stages before things run smoothly. The stages (Tuckman and Jensen, 1977) that can be anticipated are:

- forming – where the members of the team meet each other and begin to make relationships;
- storming – where attempts to develop understanding lead to disagreements and differences and cause upsets and people can feel that little progress is being made;
- norming – where agreements emerge and direction is reestablished;
- performing – where the team is working at its best and achieving targets through collaboration and co-operation.

Many teams have to go backwards through this sequence many times and some spend all of their time together storming and norming without ever reaching a satisfying performance.

Life is never as simple as models might suggest, and few of us can describe experiences of teamworking that progress in an orderly fashion through such a series of stages. Leaders in teams can help people to understand what is happening and often can facilitate productive discussions when storming seems to be distracting everyone from their purpose. If emphasis is placed on the value and importance of achieving the project outcomes successfully, discussions can be kept focused about how to progress. It is usually helpful to ensure that everyone is involved in discussions about working practice because if they are not, there will be a feeling of exclusion and possibly fear of blame.

Leaders within the team can contribute to ensuring that the common commitment to achieving the objectives is reiterated and given priority. The team may have to discuss how to handle differences before such discussions can take place. If people do not have good listening skills this might have to be discussed and some simple rules adopted to ensure that the loudest do not dominate discussions. Similarly, people may have to learn how to deliver feedback or criticism in a constructive way. If this is a training need, it is important to identify it and spend time developing the necessary skills so that everyone can take part in discussions openly and constructively. It is helpful if people will agree to raise concerns in an open way and to explain their feelings. This is only possible if those chairing meetings insist on respect for individuals.

Sometimes teams can feel as though there is unfair external judgement of them, whether there is or not. Leaders can encourage teams to be more proactive in making their own judgements about progress in project working. Regular review meetings can be held to review successes as well as problem areas and the team can be encouraged to identify learning from its developing experience.

## MANAGING YOURSELF

Although managers and leaders can share the successes of the team and enjoy the interactions when things go well, there are often times when they feel distant from the team and lacking in support themselves, particularly when they are supporting very 'needy' individuals and teams. In large projects those who are in team-leading positions can meet together and form a small team for mutual support. When a person is leading and managing a smaller project, it is important to think about where personal support can be found. In some cases the relationship with the sponsor or senior managers may supply that support. In other cases it might be worth asking a senior manager or a peer with more or different experience to be your mentor. Sessions with a mentor can be used to review not only how the project is progressing but also to reflect on your own actions and the reactions that each provoked. It can also be helpful to keep a personal journal and to note what actions you take and what reactions these produce to help you to learn more about your impact on others.

## REFERENCES

Tuckman, B. and Jensen, M. (1977) 'Stages of small group development revisited', Groups and Organizational Studies, Vol. 2, pp. 419–27.

CHAPTER 13

# MANAGING PERFORMANCE

Performance in a project is crucial to achieving objectives of the right quality within the time and costs agreed. Monitoring will reveal if areas of work are falling behind the planned schedule or if the quality of achievement is not high enough. This will inform the project manager that action needs to be taken and this is when the management of performance can become an important concern.

Expectations of performance are not always spelt out precisely in the early stages of a project. When staff are appointed to the project team there is often consideration of skills and experience, but availability often determines exactly who will be assigned to the project unless external appointments are to be made. This may mean that some of those in the project team are not able or willing to work to the standards and speed expected and required. The project manager may have to deal with staff who lack the necessary capability and staff who lack the willingness to work effectively on the project.

## PREPARING FOR GOOD PERFORMANCE

It is worth ensuring, as soon as work is able to start on the project, that staff are both able and willing to do a good job. If tasks are planned to be realistic and achievable, they can be allocated to team members in a way that allows an opportunity to discuss any concerns. Staff often have to maintain other workloads while working on projects and it may be necessary to negotiate with senior managers to ensure that project staff have sufficient time and energy to do what is required. If members of the project team face conflicting demands from other managers at your own level you may have to negotiate to resolve the risk to the project.

It may also be necessary for new skills and understanding to be developed in order to carry out new tasks. It is not always possible to recruit staff for a project using a detailed person specification. Staff are sometimes allocated simply because they have some spare time, but they may not have the competence to carry out the project tasks. The manager of a project may have to arrange for training and support, whether or not this was anticipated in the initial planning. In some cases, it may be necessary to make changes to staffing appointments to reduce the need for additional training and support. In other situations the development needs might be viewed as an opportunity presented by the project. Staff development might be addressed without additional resources being allocated to the project if the needs that have emerged are ones that routine training and development provision can address and if the additional competence gained will be of long-term use to the organisation.

In allocating roles and responsibilities when project staff are drawn from routine work, it is important to consider the levels of responsibility and authority that staff normally hold within the organisation. It is rarely successful to create a structure in which the usual lines of responsibility and accountability are reversed! For example, if you want a senior functional expert to contribute to one particular aspect of a project, this person may become very frustrated if placed in a role that is restricted by someone who lacks ability as their team leader. It may be possible to remove the more senior people from the team structure and create an advisory role to enable them to contribute the necessary knowledge and experience.

Project staff need the skills and experience to do the job required, but for the project to succeed they also need to want to do it well. The conditions in which staff work and the relationships between people always have an impact on performance and can help to create a positive climate. A project manager is often able to influence conditions and culture. There is an opportunity to develop a project culture of collaboration towards a successful goal. The boundaried nature of a project makes it possible to create a positive culture even in an environment where the culture does not always support the work of the organisation. It is often possible in a project to emphasise the positive aspects of the environment in which the project is located.

## MANAGING THE PERFORMANCE OF TEAMS IN A PROJECT

Once a team has formed, it begins to have an identity that is different from that of the individuals who are part of the team. Teams that share common values, have a sense of purpose and have developed ways of working together can be confident and powerful in achieving objectives. In health and social care settings much of the work cannot be achieved without working in teams. This can be both an advantage and a problem in a project. When teams are focused on achieving the objectives of the project, the energy can drive outstanding achievements, often beyond the expectations of individual team members.

When a team is focused on matters other than the project, however, energy can be dissipated and performance mediocre or distinctly unsatisfactory.

A project manager needs to be able to work with both scenarios. A very successful and high-achieving team still needs some support and attention. The work of the team still has to be organised and supervised and the level of performance acknowledged. A high-performing team may be motivated in several different ways and it is usually important to ensure that those rewards continue to be available if the team performance is to be maintained. Much of the satisfaction that can be gained in working in an effective project team derives from the sense of being identified with the team, feeling that your contribution is valued and that the work is worthwhile. Often individual members of a team will have very different interests and backgrounds, but will find it very satisfying to work with others who can bring a different expertise and understanding to the work. For example, a team of people collaborating to address teenage pregnancy might include social workers, teachers, GPs, health visitors, health promotion specialists and parents. The glue that would keep the team together in this project would be the purpose of the project and the potential satisfaction of making a contribution that could help to address a problem that concerns them all.

When a team is not performing effectively there could be a number of different reasons for the problem. In many cases this happens because members of the team encounter something that presents a barrier to their effective performance. This may be because they do not have the necessary skills and expertise, they may lack effective leadership or they may not want to work collaboratively. They may have encountered a problem that has stopped their work. They may simply not understand what is required of them. These are all performance management issues that can be addressed by a project manager.

## MANAGING RELATIONSHIPS AND CONFLICT

In some projects, several different types of teams may have different types of work to complete. The relationships between these teams and their team leaders can have a profound influence on the project, with the potential either to enhance smooth working or to cause damaging disruption. If the work of one team is dependent on the timing or quality of a previous team there is potential for conflict if anything goes wrong.

## ACTIVITY 13.1

*Allow 10 minutes.*

Think back to projects in which you have had a part. From your experience, note some of the ways in which you have seen teams add value to a project and some ways in which projects can be disrupted by unco-operative teamwork.

How a team can add value:

1 ____________________

2 ____________________

3 ____________________

4 ____________________

5 ____________________

How a team can disrupt:

1 ____________________

2 ____________________

3 ____________________

4 ____________________

5 ____________________

Value can be added at any stage of a project if teams focus on delivering the best that they can to their service users. In some cases this may be another team who develop the project on the basis of the first team's work. As with any customers, finding out more about what they really want and delivering the best that can be produced within the scope and budget of the project will add value. Teams that achieve all that is required of them within the resource limitations and hand over their part of the project helpfully also add value. Value can be added by using the learning from working on the project to improve working practices. New skills can be developed through project work, including skills in teamworking, supervision, coaching and peer support. You have probably thought of many other ways in which value can be added.

Teams also have considerable power to disrupt. They can delay work so that their tasks are not completed on time and they can work carelessly and produce work of a poor quality. They can allow personal interactions to cause conflict and stress. They can adopt attitudes that present a poor image of the organisation to external stakeholders. They can simply behave badly.

Unco-operative behaviour is normally addressed informally and face to face in the first instance. If behaviour continues to disrupt progress, however, more formal procedures will be needed. It might be necessary to establish a framework for performance management within the project. Many of the essentials are already in the plan, so it would not be difficult to assign specific objectives to individuals to detail the contribution that they are expected to make to their team's work and the outcomes that the work must achieve.

Conflict is a risk to the success of the project. You can manage this risk as you would any other type of risk – in a controlled manner. The management process is vital from the beginning to the end – identify the risks and analyse them, develop a risk mitigation plan and then monitor the risks.

**Example 13.1 – Risks from conflict**

An experienced project manager was discussing his experience of conflict becoming a risk in projects. He said, 'It is inevitable that conflict will develop at some stage in any project team composed of people with different personalities, backgrounds, experiences and specialist skills. Interpersonal conflict may arise where people do not want to get along because of different specialisms, racial prejudices, ethics, morals and the like. Typical causes of conflict include breakdown in communications, conflicting objectives and lack of trust. Ambition, jealousy and simply the wrong "chemistry" are not unusual. There is often fear of change, or fear that some inadequacy or failure will be exposed.'

Many approaches can be taken to reduce the possibility that conflict will damage the project. Staff can be asked to work together in an initial team building workshop to identify any conflicts that they can predict might arise. The risk of conflict is strong wherever there is personal interaction in an essential channel of communication. When these are likely to arise from specialist approaches or different professional concerns, the team members may be much more aware of the dangers than the project manager. If the team is involved in identifying the risks and preparing contingency plans, this can become a positive contribution to effective working across specialist and professional boundaries.

The risk of conflict will not disappear even if it is discussed and understood. The project manager will still need to consider what action can be taken if conflict develops. A project manager needs to be alert to signs of conflict. These will include clashes of interests and raised voices, although sometimes it will be less obvious if people feel frustrated or blocked from voicing opinions and may only be evident if individuals become reluctant to be involved in areas of work.

There are five useful approaches that a project manager might take to manage conflict when it develops:

1 Allow the conflict. If the conflict seems to be useful in helping to bring important issues to the surface you may decide to allow it to proceed. If people seem to be accepting that differences of opinion need to be expressed and considered, it is probably best to encourage open discussion and to work with those involved to identify solutions.
2 Smooth and support. It may also be possible to leave conflict to run its course if the cause is temporary and the situation will soon change, although you may have to be sympathetic and offer some temporary support to those who are particularly uncomfortable.
3 Prevent conflict. Sometimes it is possible to predict potential conflict and take action to prevent it from happening. To do this you have to know your team members well and take time to think through how you expect the situation to develop.
4 Contain conflict. Allow the conflict but prevent it from spreading beyond the area of work where it is useful or tolerated and not causing damage.
5 Reduce or eliminate the conflict. This will usually require the manager to take action to change the situation in some way.

Making changes in the organisation of the project or the roles and responsibilities of staff may help to reduce the opportunity for conflict.

Sometimes the causes of conflict are structural and a manager can reorganise things to reduce the potential for conflict. It might be possible to improve communications or even to substitute a member of staff if this becomes necessary. At worst, if it is not possible to manage conflict informally, it is possible that more formal procedures like grievance or disciplinary actions will become necessary.

As the project progresses, circumstances may change and different pressures may encourage competition or collaboration. A project manager can notice the dynamics that change and develop and can be prepared to intervene if necessary.

## MAKING REQUIREMENTS EXPLICIT

Performance requirements need to be explicit if the performance of the project team is to be measured against a standard. It is much easier to identify whether performance is at the levels expected if standards are set. Ideally, the standards of performance expected will be discussed and agreed with teams and individuals in the early stages of the project.

One of the easiest approaches to setting standards is to write objectives for each task area. These can be translated into objectives for each individual. This approach enables differences for individual contributions to be built into the cascaded objectives and for expert contributions to be identified. It also provides an overview of what is required for each task and can help to ensure that all the aspects of each task are considered and responsibility assigned for each separate area of work.

Ideally, standards of performance will be agreed with each team and individual alongside agreement about how the work will be monitored. If these are discussed fully it should also be possible to identify any potential barriers to effective performance. This will alert the project manager to potential problems and allow time for some consideration about how the issues might be addressed.

It is not always easy to set clear objectives for jobs, particularly when they support other activities. Jobs that have substantial emphasis on liaising, co-ordinating or facilitating are difficult to describe in terms of what will be achieved, but the contribution to the achievement of the team is important. It might be helpful to involve other members of the team in developing a description of the performance that is required. This process can help to develop the collaboration that will be necessary to enable smooth co-ordination.

In developing objectives for each team and individual, try also to identify the type of evidence that will demonstrate that the objectives have been achieved. This will make it much easier to comment on the work of individuals and teams when necessary and will also provide the means by which reviews can be held if performance seems to be less than satisfactory.

## ENSURING THAT THE TEAM HAVE THE NECESSARY SKILLS AND EXPERIENCE

It is not unusual for a project manager to find that some training is necessary even when those appointed to work on the project are skilled and experienced. The most basic need might not be considered as training, but is the time and range of activities needed to enable those involved in the project to contribute appropriately. This can often be achieved through holding planning workshops at the start of the project. Those involved can be asked to consider what training needs might be encountered so that the potential concerns can be identified at an early stage. For example, it is often necessary to offer training in use of computer software that is unfamiliar to some but that everyone will need to use.

In some ways, a project manager can consider the training needs as a microcosm of the usual training procedures in an organisation. Training is usually focused to ensure that each individual has the skills and knowledge necessary to enable them to perform effectively in their job. This is very important when performance is to be assessed against a specific expectation. In a project, the expectations are specific in terms of what has to be achieved by a particular time and within estimated costs. There is also an expectation about the quality of work.

All project staff will need some training. The project begins a period that is not dissimilar to that of an induction for new employees. People need to be informed about the conditions of employment and how they will be paid. They need to know to whom they are accountable and where to go for information or help. Introductions will be needed, possibly a walk around the accommodation of the project, and workshops will be needed to familiarise everyone with the plans and the part that they are expected to play in achieving the objectives. Health and safety training will usually be needed if staff are working in unfamiliar surroundings or carrying out unfamiliar activities. Questions may need to be resolved about who receives development opportunities and who does not if time and funding are limited. Decisions therefore have to be made about who should be included and for what reasons. Employers are required by law not to discriminate on the grounds of gender, marital status, race or disability when making decisions about training opportunities. It is also good practice not to discriminate on the grounds of age.

More individual training might be offered if it is necessary and if it has been funded as an activity necessary for the project to succeed. It may be training specific to the requirements of the project, possibly because staff are required to do something in a different way or to use different materials or equipment. The amount of training that you can offer in a project depends on the length of the project and the amount of training that an individual needs to be able to complete the tasks required. Training is not the answer to everything, but is often important in bringing performance up to the required level. There may be people who have been appointed to the project team without appropriate skills and experience who may not be able to improve in time even if training is offered during the project.

## DEVELOPING COLLABORATION

The nature of the task in a project can affect the extent to which team performance is necessary. If the task is fairly simple and members of the team are experienced in performing similar tasks, they may be able to work effectively with only good communications and co-operation. As the task becomes more complex, the need for more sophisticated teamwork becomes more evident. When it is difficult to understand what is needed before action can be taken, people become frustrated and anxious about progress and the need for management of the teamwork becomes greater.

When team members listen to each other, respect different points of view, share information and will collaborate and negotiate, there is usually enough teamwork to complete the tasks of a project. It may not be as much fun for the individuals concerned as it can be when there is a real sense of being part of an effective team, but objectives can be successfully achieved.

It becomes more difficult to work together when the levels of risk increase. In a difficult situation when no-one knows what sort of expertise is required or when opinions differ, it can be difficult for individuals who express views that are not popular with the majority. If individuals feel isolated by their views they may stop offering different suggestions and their contributions will be lost to the team. Sometimes this can be managed through leadership in the team, but sometimes the project manager may have to intervene. For example, the project manager could discuss with the group the benefits of ensuring that problems be considered from a wide range of perspectives and encourage them to set rules for occasions where they encounter differences. When the whole group is committed to achieving the objectives of the project this can be effective. If there is one member of the group whose behaviour prevents others from working collaboratively, that individual may have to be dealt with separately.

It is often very important to hear from individuals in a team because of the particular blend of knowledge, skills and experience they bring. A person who feels that they have much less experience or expertise than others in the group might find it difficult to contribute and may need to be supported and encouraged.

**Example 13.2 – Sharing knowledge in the project team**

I was working with the project team that were closing an old building that housed a small number of people with learning difficulties and relocating them into other local facilities. We were under time pressure and had a meeting where we moved very quickly through the plans to move each individual into his or her new home. All of the homes had been inspected recently and we had identified where there was spare capacity that we could use. The social worker in the team had mentioned that we should make provision for people to make a personal choice. Most of the others thought that this could be done by the care workers in the home once the number to go to each new location had been appropriately allocated.

When the care workers started to discuss the arrangements with the residents, there were so many issues that we hadn't considered. There were family connections that meant that people couldn't be separated, friends and social connections, some with similar interests or needs – all sorts of things that influenced the grouping.

In the end we had to hold another meeting with the care workers and the information that they had gathered and start from the other end of things. We sorted out what groupings the residents wanted to retain and then found accommodation for each group.

We should have listened to the concerns of the social worker much earlier but she said that she thought that she shouldn't say things that would slow the meeting down when everyone else seemed to know what they were doing.

There is a great deal of emphasis today on modernising service provision in health and care and we can all expect to be working in more interdisciplinary and inter-professional teams. People with different perspectives will have to collaborate more often. People will be expected to be flexible in taking on different roles in different groups. Those managing projects in health and social care will have to cope with the difficulties that arise, but the gains in achieving successful project outcomes that surmount unhelpful boundaries can far outweigh the problems.

## DEALING WITH POOR PERFORMANCE

It is much easier to spot poor performance if clear standards for performance have been set. If you suspect that an individual is under-performing, it is important to think carefully before raising the issue with the person concerned. The questions you might ask yourself are:

- What am I concerned about, exactly?
- What evidence do I have?
- Might there be an impact from the project context in which the performance is happening?
- Are there any factors that may be affecting the situation, such as inadequate equipment, stress or incompatible priorities?
- How important is this problem?
- What is its impact on patients or service users?
- Does it harm our collective effectiveness as a team?
- Are my concerns important enough or legitimate enough to merit intervention?
- Am I concerned about isolated incidents or small behavioural quirks that may not be important to others?
- Is there any indication that my concerns are shared (or not shared) by others?
- Would it be helpful to share my perceptions with the person involved? Would it help him or her to understand how he or she is being seen, and provide an opportunity to clarify some mutual expectations?

If you want to raise the issue with the person involved, ensure that you have details of the standards that were set for the performance and any evidence that you have that these standards were not being met. If you start by discussing this openly without accusing the person involved, further information might be offered and a solution might become evident.

The reasons for poor performance can usually be classified into one of three categories:

1 A person doesn't understand what he or she has to do. This may be because the expectations have not been thoroughly discussed.

2 He or she is not capable of doing it consistently. This might be addressed by providing further training.
3 He or she is knowingly not doing what is required. This implies that the individual will not conform to expectations and their performance may become a disciplinary matter.

Often, expectations about general behaviour should be made explicit if employees must comply with them. These include rules about attendance and absence, time-keeping, health and safety, compliance with instructions and confidentiality of information.

## DISCIPLINARY PROCEDURES

Projects differ in how disciplinary procedures take place. If a project is taking place within the usual procedures of an organisation, then the usual disciplinary rules are likely to apply. If a project is inter-organisational, it is important to establish which disciplinary procedures will be used. Staff who are appointed to the project team should be informed of the grievance and disciplinary procedures so that they know exactly what policies will be used if there is a serious disagreement.

Any expectations of employees should be explicit, perhaps in the form of policies or conditions of work. These might include details of what is expected in each of the following areas:

- times of work;
- absence and arrangements for sick leave;
- health and safety and the responsibilities of the individual;
- procedures for use of the organisation's facilities and limits on personal use;
- equal opportunities and discrimination;
- disclosure of confidential information;
- compliance with instructions;
- how expenses should be claimed;
- rules about accepting gifts or hospitality;
- rules governing contact with the media.

The overall disciplinary policy must explain the procedure that will be taken if the rules are broken.

Employment law places a legal obligation on any employer with 20 or more employees to include, within written terms and conditions of employment, details of:

- any disciplinary rules which apply to the employee, and
- the name of the person whom the employee should notify if dissatisfied with any disciplinary decision.

The standard of work of an employee can also be a matter for disciplinary action if the person appears to be refusing to comply with expectations. This is often difficult to prove and it is very important for a manager who thinks that disciplinary action for this reason will be necessary to comply with the procedures of their organisation or to seek help if they are unsure of the procedures. It is very important to establish that any employee who is accused of poor performance was informed of the standards expected and of any conditions attached to a probationary period.

A disciplinary procedure describes the process by which disciplinary matters are managed. Its purpose is to ensure that an employee who has breached the required standards of behaviour or work performance (but not grossly so) is given a fair opportunity to improve. Although it may eventually lead to the dismissal of the employee, this is not its main purpose. One of the main areas to come under scrutiny, should a case eventually end up at an industrial tribunal, will be the disciplinary procedure itself: whether it was followed properly, and whether the employer's actions and penalties were fair and reasonable.

As a project manager, you should know what the disciplinary procedure is and ensure that you comply with it. You should also be aware that in the health service some groups of staff, such as doctors, dentists and nurses, may be governed by their national terms and conditions of service regarding disciplinary matters. You will almost certainly want to take advice from your human resources department or senior managers.

## GRIEVANCE PROCEDURES

Grievance procedures provide a formal mechanism through which individual employees or groups can bring their concerns or complaints to the attention of their employer and have them addressed. The procedures deal with problems arising in the workplace that could adversely affect a member of staff's mental or physical well-being, or his or her ability to perform to the standard of work expected. Employment law requires any employer with 20 or more employees to include in written terms and conditions of employment the name of the person to whom an employee can take a grievance and details of the way in which a grievance will be handled. An employee can take out a grievance if treated in a way that he or she feels breaks the rules of law, contract, or the 'accepted custom and practice' of the way things are done if it works to his or her disadvantage.

Most people want to perform well and managers are not often involved in either grievance or disciplinary procedures. The procedures are there to provide fair ways of handling situations in which things go wrong. Although most people would prefer not to have to move into formal procedures, they are there to enable a fair process and it is sometimes necessary for a project manager to take responsibility for ensuring that the procedures are followed. It is essential that you do not start to take any action until you are sure that you know the procedures thoroughly. Before taking action you should investigate the problem thoroughly and listen to as many different points of view as possible. You will need to keep records of the actions that you have taken and you will need to provide evidence if the disciplinary action moves into the formal process. In most cases it is enough to remind people of the procedure and the agreements that were made, but occasionally the procedures have to be enacted and followed carefully before a decision can be reached.

The time-scales and objectives of a project usually dictate the extent to which poor performance can be tolerated. Often, less time is available before action must be taken than there is in day-to-day work. A project manager always has to keep the demands of the project as the main focus when making decisions about what action to take.

CHAPTER 14

# COMPLETING THE PROJECT

As a project nears its completion, the focus moves on from implementation activities to ensuring that all the deliverables have been handed over to the appropriate recipients. Deliverables are not always tangible products and handover may require support or training to enable the use of new processes or technology. Delivery of the outcomes will vary according to the purpose and objectives of the project, but all the outcomes and deliverables need to be either formally handed over, or accounted for if anything is missing.

## HANDOVER AND DELIVERY

The deliverables of a project are usually listed at an early stage of planning. At this stage arrangements should be made for any conditions that are necessary for the transfer of responsibility to be completed. For example, delicate equipment would not normally be handed over until there is a safe place for it to be installed ready for use. Handover is usually a formal procedure where the person responsible for accepting the delivery checks everything and 'signs off' the item as complete and of the agreed quality. This process ensures that there is no dispute about whether the project outcomes have been completed.

**Example 14.1 – Relocating a joint service**

A health service manager was leading a project to relocate a joint social services and health care clinic and advisory service into part of a new tower block. The project was complex because the new location required different working practices, particularly for some of the regular services. Handover of all of the physical aspects of the project, including installation of new partition walls, furnishing and equipment, was easily managed as each item could be signed off by the relevant manager. It was more difficult to make arrangements for the services, including cleaning, electricity, toilets, lifts and use of the shared ground-floor reception area.

After researching how these had been managed in other projects, he devised a chart of required services and worked with managers of the new joint service area to identify the standards required of each contracted support service. He then wrote a 'Service Level Agreement' for each service to be contracted, that set out what was required. The Service Level Agreement was a document and could be 'signed off' as a deliverable from the project, but it included details of the process by which the joint service managers would contract and regularly review the services.

In some projects there are handovers before the conclusion of the project. These are often between different teams working on sequential tasks. Although it is not necessary to insist on a formal delivery, some record should be made in case a dispute arises about where responsibility lies. In some projects a complete project objective is handed over at an early stage. For example, a building site may be handed over before any demolition or building work can begin. The agreements governing the condition in which a site is handed over can be very complex because some problems can cause significant delay. For example, it is a serious problem if asbestos is found during demolition because specialist services will need time to make the site safe before any work can continue.

Handovers should have been identified as key stages on the Gantt chart. If the project involves the preparation and handover of a physical object, there may be a number of contributing components. The project plan will have identified the various elements and will include details of handover arrangements for each stage if there is a sequence of tasks. The schedule will identify the sequence in which tasks need to be completed. Hopefully, the risk register will have identified the risks associated with each handover and a contingency plan will have been made for each major risk.

When the outcome is a physical product, it is usually fairly easy to define the acceptance criteria. It is more difficult to write acceptance criteria for projects that have developed a new process or service. If the objectives of the project have been written carefully, the key expectations will be detailed in a way that helps to identify exactly what should be included in the handover. It is much better to discuss this in the early stages of planning than to find that there are different expectations in the final stages of the project. If new items are added to the deliverables at a late stage, it is very difficult to complete the project within the budget and time-scales that have been allowed.

If training or support is necessary before the client or sponsor can make full use of the project outcomes, this should have been anticipated and built into the project plans. Accepting additional tasks in the late stages can be very difficult because staff allocated to the project team will often have made arrangements to move directly on to different work after the completion date of their contracts.

Often a number of small tasks or non-urgent details are outstanding as the delivery date approaches. The team leader or project manager should ensure that someone is responsible for the completion of each item and that they have the means to do the necessary work.

## DELIVERING WITH STYLE

You can deliver the outcomes agreed with the minimum of fuss or celebration or you can deliver with style. Many of us will have been delighted with a beautifully wrapped gift. A project that meets the outcomes on time and within the budget will be well received, but if it is well presented it will enhance the impression of professionalism and care in completing the work.

Each delivery offers an opportunity to please the client with presentation of a successful outcome. For example, when a new suite of rooms that have been fitted out for use as offices are handed over to the client, there is only one chance to make a first impression! The project could be completed with furniture assembled and in place, but carpets may be left covered in dust and wrappings left in a pile by the main entrance, waiting for different contractors to clear it away. How much better it would be if someone spent a few minutes vacuuming the carpet and clearing away the debris. Even better, if someone placed a few vases of fresh flowers on the shelves or desks. Presentation is about creating an impression. There is an opportunity with the handover events of a project to create a favourable or unfavourable impression.

## PLANNING FOR A SUCCESSFUL CONCLUSION

A successful project may conclude with a satisfied client, pleased stakeholders and a proud but sad team!

The successful completion of a project is the purpose of all of the effort and work, but the end of a project is often a sad event for those who have enjoyed working together in the project team. As the team will disband quickly once the project activities are complete, it is worth thinking about holding a celebration while it is still intact. Celebration of success demonstrates confidence in the project. A concluding celebration can be planned in from an early date. Some teams celebrate each milestone review!

Celebratory events usually motivate the team, giving momentum in the later stages of a long project. A news-sheet and public announcements can also be effective. Celebrations and announcements give an opportunity to acknowledge the efforts of the team and contribute to keeping morale high.

**Example 14.2 – Closing with an event**

The project was the development of a joint commissioning strategy for several community services. The outcome of the project was the launch of the jointly agreed strategic plan that would be implemented by the joint commissioning team.

The team were anxious to ensure that service users understood the benefits that would flow from the strategy and held a number of different types of publicity event. They held workshops with staff from each of the relevant service areas to explore how the strategy would require them to work differently and to develop understanding of the potential benefits for their areas of work. The joint commissioning team took care to ensure that staff from all of the contributing services were fully informed about the new strategy so that they would act as good ambassadors for the developments.

The new team issued publicity releases to the media and held a public meeting at which the details were announced and the team answered questions. Anxieties and potential problems were acknowledged and the measures that would be taken to reduce risk were discussed. The new strategy was received with interest and the openness of the new team was welcomed.

## CLOSING THE PROJECT

The closing stage of a project needs planning in a similar way to earlier activities. It is a shame if an otherwise successful project is left in a messy condition when the members of the project team have to move quickly on to other areas of work. Once the main purpose of the project has been achieved, the tasks of closure can seem like rather tedious housekeeping. If the project team have been enjoying the work, you might have to make sure that they all stop working on the project once everything that was part of the agreement has been delivered. It is always necessary to ensure that payments for time and expenses are completed and discontinued. The project manager will also usually be involved in arranging the final review or evaluation.

All projects generate documentation and the project manager should ensure that records that might be needed again are stored safely and can be retrieved. Documents that confirm that all contractual obligations were completed are kept along with the project plans, budgets and relevant staff records. The minutes of all major meetings are kept so that agreements that were made can be reviewed and it is also usual to keep all versions of the project plan with the notes that relate to changes made.

The financial aspects of a project need special attention in the closing stages. The manager of the project usually has responsibility for the budget and needs to ensure that all expenditure is accounted for in the final statement of expenditure. This stage is particularly important if the client has authorised any expenditure that was not part of the original estimate. Clients do not always remember or realise the extent to which additional small items of expenditure can add up to substantial sums in the final analysis. A clear record of purchases should be made, shown through orders, delivery notes and payments made against invoices. Any discrepancies should be explained and evidence provided wherever possible. In some cases it might be necessary to hold a formal financial audit. The financial accounting must be completed and some arrangements made for any outstanding unpaid invoices and any remaining assets or materials.

## CLOSURE CHECKLISTS

In a complex project it can be helpful to think of the closure activities as a small project in themselves and to plan for them as a distinct set of tasks. You will probably want to make a detailed list of what needs to be done.

---

### ACTIVITY 14.1

*Allow 5 minutes.*

Make notes of the key headings that you think should feature on a project closure check-list.

______________________________

______________________________

______________________________

______________________________

______________________________

You might have listed key deliverables and associated tasks to ensure that the purpose of the project had been achieved. Another main heading might include all the 'housekeeping' elements of completing staff-related matters, financial records and any outstanding materials and equipment used. You might have suggested a reminder to stop all activities, supplies and processes related to the project activities. You might also have considered having headings that would determine who should carry out each task and identify the date by which each task should be completed.

---

As in all other aspects of managing a project, management of closure can be planned and the tasks can be delegated. One benefit of preparing a detailed list is that responsibilities for each task can be assigned with dates to indicate when actions can be started and when they should be completed. There may be scheduling issues even at this stage to ensure that tasks are sequenced and prioritised if necessary.

A closure list is likely to include the following tasks, but each project will have different features to consider. Suggested areas include:

- handover completed for all deliverables;
- client or sponsor has signed off all deliverables;
- final project reports are complete;
- all financial processes and reports are complete and budget is closed;
- project review is complete and comments recorded;
- staff performance evaluations and reports are completed;
- staff employment on project is terminated;
- all supply contracts and processes are terminated;
- all project site operations are closed down and accommodation used for the project is handed back;
- equipment and materials are disposed of in an appropriate way;
- the project completion is announced (internal, external and public relations contacts);
- the project records are completed and stored appropriately.

If the manager of a project moves on to another assignment before all of these tasks are complete, a list of this type can be used as the agenda for a discussion about how to hand over responsibilities for effective completion of the project.

## DISMANTLING THE TEAM

The end of a project can be quite an emotional experience for team members who have worked together for some time, particularly if close bonds have developed. The schedule will have indicated when team members complete their tasks, so in many projects staff move to other work before the project is completed. Even if staff are not moved into other work, many of the project team members will plan their own futures in relation to the anticipated completion of the project. For some there will be a sense of loss, but others may be excited by new opportunities offered in their next work assignment. In some cases new opportunities will have arisen as a result of skills and experience that have been gained as a result of working on the project.

The manager of a project has some obligations to staff who have worked for some time on a project. You can allow time to have a closure interview with each member of staff so that their contribution can be formally acknowledged and recorded. Many staff will need help to recognise the skills and experience that they have gained and to gather evidence of their contribution and achievements. Many staff would welcome a signed record of their achievements and some will need references to progress to their next jobs. Others might welcome support in reviewing their careers and in considering directions that may have been made possible by their involvement in the project. At this stage, the focus for the team will be to disengage from the project, owning their contribution and relinquishing their collective identity. Effective debriefing can help to maintain their commitment through to the end.

The timing of project closure may be a delicate matter, as some staff will leave before the project is fully finished and others will not have jobs to go to. The project is not finished until the closure has been managed and it is helpful if the people managing these final activities are not worried about their own futures. Once again, planning well in advance can reduce the stress of the final stages of the project.

## PROJECT DRIFT

When one project leads into another without a clear break or when extra tasks that were not identified at the beginning are added to a project, this is called project drift. Ideally, significant changes should be treated separately as a follow-on project. If the project is allowed to drift into provision of additional outcomes, they may not be properly resourced because they were not included in the plans at an early enough stage. Project drift can have adverse consequences for the motivation of the project team and difficulties may be encountered if staff are expected to take on additional work once their planned involvement in the project is complete.

**Example 14.3 – A drifting project**

A community centre that had housed a local authority youth club and services for young people was to become empty when the services transferred to accommodation in a new local shopping centre. The empty building was to be handed over to the community association to pay the full costs of their own use and maintenance of the building.

The transfer of the youth services out of the building took place as planned. However, the building was not handed over immediately because the local authority decided to use it to provide emergency accommodation because there had been increased media attention highlighting the number of homeless young people sleeping in the streets.

The project manager who was responsible for the transfer of the building to the local community association had to return to other work. To avoid project drift, a new manager was appointed to deal with the emergency use of the building and the original project was closed as the youth club and services had been successfully transferred to their new accommodation. The community development initiative was put on hold with a view to appointing a new project manager to complete the task when the building became available again.

If project drift leaves aspects of the project unfinished or continuing without a planned completion time, it may be impossible to carry out the normal closure activities. It might be possible, and helpful, to consider closing off the phase of the project that has been achieved. For example, you might hold a review to establish what could be considered finished and what needs to remain in place to allow the next stages to progress. It is often helpful to use such a review to close off what has been done so far. This may then allow a fresh start, to approach the new possibilities as if this were the beginning of a new project. Taking this approach helps stakeholders to return to the fundamental questions about the purpose and goals of the project, to define the anticipated outcomes and to set new boundaries for the time-scale, budget and quality requirements.

CHAPTER 15

# EVALUATING THE PROJECT

Evaluation involves making a judgement about value. Evaluation usually takes place at the end of the project, but one can be held during a project if a need is perceived for something more substantial than a review. Sometimes evaluations are held quite a long time after the completion of a project to see whether the long-term aims were achieved effectively.

If it is to be effective, evaluation needs to be focused in some way so that it is clear what is to be judged and what the considerations are likely to be.

## ACTIVITY 15.1

*Allow 10 minutes.*

Make a note of what you might evaluate at the end of a project.

You might want to carry out an overall performance evaluation to consider the economy and efficiency of the performance through which the outcomes were achieved or not against the planning process. There might also be evaluation of inputs into the project, to review whether the resources were adequate in quality and quantity for the job. You would usually evaluate the outcomes to identify the extent to which all of the intended outcomes were achieved. The outcomes might be wider in scope than the objectives if the purpose of the project was to carry out a change through the achievement of a group of objectives. This might review the overall effectiveness of the outcomes and might also seek to identify any unintended outcomes. Of course, an evaluation might be planned to consider several of these factors at once.

---

It is very important to determine the purpose of an evaluation before setting up a process. Evaluations are often held to report on the value of outcomes achieved in relation to the value of investment of resources to achieve that outcome. Where value is concerned, opinions often vary and one of the key questions to ask at an early stage is who should carry out the evaluation and whose opinions should be taken into account. Evaluations have to be reported in some way and often make recommendations for future projects as well as reporting on the one being evaluated. In this sense, often a lot of learning can be captured by carrying out an evaluation so that future projects can benefit from that previous experience.

## EVALUATION DURING A PROJECT

In the early stages of a large project it might be appropriate to carry out an evaluation to ensure that the inputs planned are of a sufficiently high quality and quantity to enable the objectives to be achieved. This can be particularly important if competition to be awarded valuable contracts will be significant. If potential contractors are very anxious to win a contract, they might try to do so by offering the lowest price or the quickest completion date. This might be attractive to those responsible for making the choice, but if the contractor proves to be unable to deliver what was promised, the project will suffer. Those evaluating tenders need to be able to anticipate the budget and timing necessary for a particular piece of work in order to make an effective evaluation of tender bids – the cheapest is not necessarily the best, nor is the one that seems to promise an impossibly fast completion.

Even when a tendering process is carried out carefully, with care to ensure that the selection results in a partnership that will be successful for everyone, it is impossible to predict all the areas of potential risk. Some contingency might be agreed, but many contracts also provide for a process to negotiate liability for additional costs if these arise unexpectedly.

There may also be an evaluation to determine whether the project is going in the right direction, particularly if a change in environmental conditions may indicate the need for a change in the strategic direction of the organisation. It might be necessary in that case to realign the project so that the outcomes contribute to the new direction. In some cases, it may be necessary to abort the project if it is no longer appropriate or likely to make a useful contribution.

Incorporating an early evaluation as part of the project plan (*formative evaluation*) can considerably enhance the outcomes. However, one of the most important characteristics that differentiate a project from wider change management is its boundaried nature. If change is anticipated during the life of the project there will be implications for all aspects of the management of the project. If it is to be included, formative evaluation should be an integral part of the design of the project. It can facilitate a more organic change process, with testing and refining built in as the project progresses. However, it can increase the complexity of a project because of the need to synchronise an extra set of deadlines that relate to carrying out the evaluation. It will also add new items to the risk log, particularly the risk of delays. A formative evaluation that results in decisions to make more significant changes to the project may increase the time-scale or the budget or present requirements to meet additional quality measures.

## EVALUATION AT THE END OF A PROJECT

Many different types of evaluation may take place at the end of a project. The most usual evaluation is to determine the extent to which the project outcomes have been achieved. This is often carried out in a meeting of the sponsor, key stakeholders and the project team leaders, sometimes informed by reports from key perspectives. An evaluation of this nature may be the final stage in completion of the project and the main purpose is usually to ensure that the project has met all of the contracted expectations and can be 'signed off' as complete. A different type of evaluation may be held to review the process with the purpose of learning from experience. This is often done by comparing the project plan with what actually happened to identify all the variations that occurred, both in terms of processes and outcomes. The purpose in this approach is to draw out the key lessons in terms of how to avoid such variations in future projects and how to plan more effectively for contingencies.

An evaluation based on the information gained through monitoring may be held at the end of the project as a final *summative evaluation*. This is a process through which to identify:

- whether the project objectives have all been achieved;
- what aspects of the project went well;
- what aspects went less well;
- what you would do differently next time.

The aim of this type of evaluation is to understand the reasons for success or failure and thus to learn from the experience in order to improve on performance in future. At the end of a project it is possible to evaluate the extent to which each stage of the project went to plan and to explore the implications of any deviations from the original plan. The implications might reveal that planning could have been more detailed or accurate, that there were obstacles that had not been predicted, that estimates had been inaccurate or that other aspects of the relationship between plans and actions could have been managed more effectively. Evaluation of the separate stages of a project is also likely to produce information that can be used to improve the management of projects in future.

Another type of evaluation that can be usefully carried out after a project is a wider consideration of the extent to which the project succeeded in achieving its purpose as a contribution to the progress of the service or organisation. This type of evaluation might be wide enough to include all recent projects held within an area of work, to investigate whether the contributions made by each were good value. It might also consider whether the value could have been increased by managing them in a different way, perhaps by linking them as part of a larger project or by splitting them into smaller projects. Although it will be too late to change what has happened, much can be learnt that can inform how future projects are defined and managed. For example, it might be found that more assistance is needed to enable project managers to estimate costs and times and that other resources from the organisation (perhaps finance, personnel or health and safety) could have helped. If projects frequently involve staff in taking the lead in managing projects it might be appropriate to develop specific training to improve how projects are managed.

The lessons learnt from evaluations can be used to inform higher level strategic planning as well as to improve management of projects.

## DESIGNING A FORMAL EVALUATION

Reviews and informal evaluations will often be sufficient, but there will be times when a formal evaluation is necessary. A formal evaluation can be both time-consuming and expensive because of the numbers of people involved and therefore it must be carefully designed and planned.

A number of decisions have to be made in designing an evaluation. The following questions will help you to begin to plan:

- What is the evaluation for?
- Who wants the evaluation?
- What is to be evaluated?
- What information will be needed?
- How and from what sources will the information be gathered?
- How will criteria for evaluation be set and by whom?
- Who will do the evaluation?
- Who will manage the process?
- How will the findings be presented?
- What use will be made of the findings?

All of these questions relate to the overall purpose in deciding to hold an evaluation and if each is considered as part of the design process, the answers will enable the process to be planned.

The purpose of the evaluation should be considered in order to identify clear aims and objectives for the process. It is helpful to decide where the boundaries of the evaluation should lie – how much or how little is to be evaluated? It can be costly and time-consuming to hold an evaluation. A cost is involved in collecting information and preparing documentation as well as in holding the necessary meetings. You might save some expense by considering the extent to which already existing information might be used.

The purpose of an evaluation determines, to some extent, who the audience for delivery of the results should be. An outcome evaluation might be for the sponsor of a project but a performance evaluation might be undertaken for a service provider part-way through a project. The nature of the audience may also determine the way in which the results of the evaluation are reported and used.

One of the key decisions in the planning stage is to decide who should carry out the evaluation. If, for example, the evaluation was of the outcome of a major project paid for by public funding, an external and independent evaluator would usually carry it out so that the results would be credible to the general public. A formal evaluation of a collaborative project might be held by a group of the key stakeholders, each able to report back to their own group or organisation. An external evaluator might be costly, but an internal evaluation will draw on time and energy that might be better devoted to carrying out the project. It is important that those conducting the evaluation should be able to understand the context and the issues that were raised in the project, but it is also important to find people who can be open and objective. This may mean seeking evaluators who did not have any direct role in the processes or outcomes of the project but who know and understand your organisation well.

In some projects in health and social care settings the choice of those who should be involved is constrained by a need for confidentiality. Although it is very important to bring a wide range of perspectives into the evaluation, it is not always appropriate for confidential information to be shared outside the small group that would normally need to access it. Involvement of service users and the general public is very important if stakeholders to projects are to be considered in evaluations of projects in health and social care, but any confidential data must be very carefully managed. There may be a number of roles to consider, including whether particular people should be involved in considering the questions or only in providing evidence.

Evaluation involves making judgements about the value of the project. Value judgements are relative and subjective and it can be very helpful to have some explicit standard against which judgements can be made. In many projects it can be difficult to make comparisons with anything similar. When there are quality standards for any of the outcomes these provide a framework that can be used, perhaps alongside targets for time-scales and resource use in achieving the necessary level of quality. Another source of comparable data might be found in benchmarks where these exist for similar activities. Benchmarks have been established for many processes and are available from industry, sector and professional bodies.

Some of the key questions to consider in carrying out an evaluation of the planning and implementation of a project are:

- Were all the objectives achieved?
- What went well and why?
- What hindered progress?
- What was helpful about the project plan?
- What was unhelpful about the project plan or hindered the work?
- Did we accurately predict the major risks and did the contingency plans work?
- Was the quality maintained at an appropriate level?
- Was the budget managed well and did we complete the project within the budget?
- Was the timing managed well and did we complete the project within the time-scale?
- Did anyone outside the project team contribute towards achieving the project?
- Did anyone or any other departments hinder the project activities?

To address these questions, you will need information from a wide range of sources. If you plan to carry out this type of evaluation it is helpful to make a plan to ensure that you collect the appropriate data when they become available, rather than expecting to find that they are still all available at the end of the project. In particular, it is usually worth recording the comments and decisions made in review meetings and in any meetings held to resolve problems that are encountered.

**Example 15.1 – Collecting information for an evaluation**

A training and consultancy organisation was contracted to provide a development programme for first-line managers in health and care services in the locality. The purpose of the programme was to increase the potential pool of senior managers. The steering group decided to plan the evaluation at an early stage in the project so that information could be collected throughout the process.

They considered how to collect data about the performance of the project in each of the three dimensions of time, cost and quality. This was to include:

- data about the planned schedules for activities and the completion times of actual events;
- data about the budget, from the estimates and initial forecasts and from the records of financial performance;

- data about quality of accommodation, equipment and any training materials used;
- data about presentation and content of the programme;
- data about the impact that the training had on performance of participants.

They recognised that there may be many different perceptions about what was delivered and how it might have been improved. In order to consider the different views, they planned to collect data from the programme providers, from participants and from the line managers of participants. Data were also to be collected from other senior managers, staff from their Human Resources department and some of the key clients of the participants.

The project team was an obvious source of data, but the planning group also decided to collect data from supporting staff, including administrative staff and other service departments that could provide perspectives on the project. Similarly, staff who managed the accommodation were also asked to provide information about how the processes were managed.

In planning the evaluation, the steering group also realised that it would be important to seek a longer-term view, perhaps six months after the conclusion of the project, to assess the extent to which it actually achieved its purpose in enabling more internal promotions.

The balance between qualitative and quantitative data is important because each can supplement the other and it is difficult to achieve an overall picture if only one type of data is used.

A number of methods can be used to collect and analyse data. Some data collection usually takes place as part of the project activities and can contribute to evaluations. For example, records kept for monitoring purposes may be used to make comparisons between activities. Records of meetings and other formal events may also provide useful data relating to the sequence of decisions made and issues discussed. Other data might be collected purely for the purposes of the evaluation. For example, interviews or questionnaires might be used to collect different views or focus groups might be used to explore issues with a group of people. Observation or role-play might be useful if data were needed about how activities are carried out.

When you are planning the data collection for an evaluation it is usual to try to obtain a range of different types of data. If only quantitative data were available you would only have information about things that could be counted. Although this is often very important, you would have no information about quality. You would want to know that the project had achieved both formal quality standards and any other expectations identified in the objectives. Opinions of those who are customers of the project are very important if you are evaluating outcomes. The views of the teams who have contributed to the project are important in evaluating the process.

The methods you choose to collect information will be influenced by the availability of resources. However, the key things to take into account are:

- the *cost* of obtaining the information in relation to its contribution to the evaluation;
- the *number of sources* from which information should be obtained if sufficient viewpoints are to be represented to ensure that the results are credible;
- the *time* it will take to obtain and analyse the information;
- the *reliability* of the information obtained;
- the *political aspects* of the process – for example, some ways of gathering information may help build up support for the evaluation.

Direct contact with those involved in the project might be the only way in which sufficient information can be obtained to make the evaluation of value.

## ANALYSING AND REPORTING THE RESULTS

When planning what data to use in the evaluation, it is helpful to consider how the data will be analysed. Usually, there is a considerable amount of data and they may be in several different forms. If you have set clear objectives, it should be possible to identify the data that are relevant in considering each issue. It is usual to consider:

- quantity, for example how much has been achieved at what cost;
- quality, was the quality appropriate and not too high or low;
- what evidence supports claims to quantity and quality;
- how the project outcome compares with alternative ways in which similar outcomes might have been achieved;
- if anything can be learnt from patterns in the evidence that can inform future projects.

It can be very time-consuming to analyse data from interviews and observations, but these approaches often collect very relevant data.

It is possible that several different evaluation reports might be prepared as part of the completion of a project. If a project was carried out as a contract, an evaluation report might be shared with the client or sponsor. There might be a different type of report if the evaluation is carried out to inform the project team's organisation about what can be learnt from their experience of this particular project. There may even be different types of evaluation reports for different stakeholders. For example, some funding bodies require reports that indicate how their funding contributed to the success of a project and they may require a report relating only to one aspect of a project. It is usually the responsibility of the manager of a project to identify the number and types of reports that are required and to ensure that they are prepared and presented appropriately.

## FOLLOW-UP TO THE REPORT

The evaluation report will often contain recommendations that suggest further actions. These recommendations need to be discussed by those who make strategic plans and further actions need to be considered. Many projects spawn other projects, particularly if they have been successful and the outcomes well received. There may be an opportunity to develop the relationship with the sponsor or client and to carry out a further similar project. There may be recommendations that relate to processes and procedures within the organisation. A project often identifies areas that need to change within organisations if they are to be able to operate flexibly to respond to external change and the increasing demand for project-working approaches.

As well as providing opportunities for individual learning, project evaluation and debriefing can be a learning experience for the organisation. This learning can be lost if insufficient time is given to thinking the process through at the end of the project. The highlights may stick in your mind, but the detail will disappear unless it is documented. In a large organisation and when projects represent very significant investment, the lessons learned from projects may well lead to changes to the organisation's policies and procedures.

CHAPTER 16

# REPORTING THE PROJECT

Projects are often of interest to a large number of people and reports about progress and achievements have to be prepared for different groups and individuals. Most of these reports are the responsibility of the project manager. Others in the team may produce reports about the current status of the project or about progress in tasks and activities, but the project manager maintains the overview. The project manager is responsible for the progress and achievements of the project and is called upon to report when required.

There might be many differences in the audiences for project reports. You may be called upon to produce a written report to go to a committee, a brief update for senior managers, a draft press briefing or notes for a public event. You might be asked to make an oral presentation, perhaps with visual aids, to an audience of Board members, to a team in your organisation, or to a large public meeting. You might be intending to write a report about managing the project to gain credit towards an academic or professional award. Each of these purposes will require a different type of preparation and format.

## WRITING A PROJECT REPORT

A project report is similar to any other business report. You have to focus on the issue that you are reporting and plan to present what the audience wants to know in a well structured and logical format. You will need to use appropriate and clear language so that they can understand what you are saying. You will have to give information about the purpose and context of the report but also to focus on aspects of the project that are particularly significant for this audience.

There are often several different project reports. When there have been a lot of different stakeholders with different hopes and concerns, it is often helpful to give information to each group in a way that meets its particular needs. It may be appropriate to use similar paragraphs to outline the purpose, background and context of the project, but the detailed information about progress or outcomes in an area of the project might be focused for the interests of a specific individual or group.

**Example 16.1 – Reporting a multifaceted project**

The purpose of the project was to develop care in the community for people with mental health problems. The project was funded from several sources, including two Health Authorities and a Regional National Health Office and had a twelve-month time-scale. More than ten Primary Health Care organisations were involved in the project alongside four Social Services Departments and several charities and voluntary organisations. A development consultancy had a research and co-ordination role, part of which included production of project reports.

Many interim reports reviewed the progress in different geographic areas. The project was arranged into six focal areas, each of which had its own objectives and schedule for developments. Each of these was run as a separate project within the whole initiative and the consultancy team supported each of the separate local teams and provided information that could be shared as events developed. Milestones were set to fit a quarterly pattern that allowed quarterly progress reports to be made about all of the projects in a newsletter form. Reports were also prepared for the funding agencies at each milestone period, giving an account of the progress against each objective and accounting for the financial expenditure at each date. Public meetings were held in each locality at the beginning of the project to invite the participation of members of the community and to inform the press and other media. The involvement of service users and carers was secured through personal contacts from both voluntary and statutory agencies.

At the end of the project a formal and detailed report was produced for the funding agencies and was made available to all of the participating organisations. A two-page information sheet that outlined the purpose and achievements in bullet points was produced in large quantities. This was made available in all the localities as a 'pick-up' newsletter to inform the general public. A media press release was prepared and distributed that gave an overview of the whole project and also reported the outcomes in each locality. This resulted in radio and television coverage of some of the outcomes including visits to some of the drop-in centres that had been established, particularly those with attractive settings and gardens.

One of the consultancy team was using her experience in the project team to contribute to study for a postgraduate award. She had contributed to the development of many of the project reports and used some of this material to develop her report for the academic award. She had to add several sections that reported on the learning gained from the experience and took a critically reflective view on the processes of the project. Several others from different local projects completed papers that were published in academic and professional journals.

Think carefully about how to report any matters that may not be welcome reading for the audience. If you encountered problems in some aspects of the work, be careful about identifying probable causes if there is an implication of blame. Consider who will read the report and how the findings might be used. It is usually better to report problems that have implications for contractual relationships in a confidential report or in a face-to-face meeting. Any problems that impede progress need to be considered and their causes addressed, but in an appropriate forum. Members of the project team and stakeholders might resent selective reporting that avoided presenting a full picture, so an appropriate balance needs to be achieved according to the context of the project.

## CHARACTERISTICS OF A GOOD REPORT

Before attempting to write, consider the purpose of the report. Most reports are written to give information, to present options in preparation for a decision or to present recommendations for action. The focus, content, style and language will be appropriate for the report's audience. The document will have a clear structure and will use headings and subheadings to guide the reader through the different sections. Spelling and grammar will be correct and the presentation will create a good impression by being tidy and businesslike. The cover will give sufficient information for a reader to see quickly what the report is about, who wrote it and when it was written. A summary will be provided and this might be written in a way that enables it to be used as a briefing sheet for a wider audience than that of the full report.

The key characteristics of a good report are:

- the purpose of the report is made clear;
- the audience for the report is identified;
- the structure of the report is clear;
- headings and subheadings act as signposts;
- care is taken over presentation, spelling and grammar;
- a summary is given;
- the focus, style and language are appropriate for the audience.

All of these elements need to be considered at the planning stage.

## STYLE, STRUCTURE AND FORMAT

There is no one right style for reports. The report with its separate title page, contents list, acknowledgements and detailed paragraph numbering might be seen as excellent in one organisation, but may be thought to be long and cumbersome in another context. You may work for an organisation that has a defined 'house style' – if so, you should follow this for reports at work, but not always if reports are to be made to external audiences. For example, a briefing prepared for a public meeting would normally be different in style from an internal management report.

Some basic elements are almost always included. For example, a basic minimum of information needs to be provided at the start of a report. This normally includes the title of the report, who it was prepared for, the author, the date and possibly the organisation name and logo. A report normally has the following sections:

- Title, author, date, and so forth on a title page.
- Contents page, listing headings, subheadings and the page numbers for each.
- Summary (sometimes called an executive summary). A one-page summary of the purpose, background and main issues addressed in the report. This will usually briefly describe how the project was carried out and note the main achievements and any recommendations that were made.
- Introduction. This usually covers the purpose of the project and briefly outlines the context.
- Background to the project. This gives whatever additional information is essential to understanding why the project was needed and how it was proposed and agreed.
- Terms of reference. This outlines the key objectives and gives any other relevant information about assumptions or constraints.
- Methods. This may report on methods of investigation or methods used to plan and implement the project. Problems encountered and overcome might be mentioned.
- Analysis. This section would be necessary only if the project had included a lot of research or investigation that necessitated some sort of interpretation or analysis, and the methods used to do that would be reported here.
- Results. This section reports the results, either of the investigation or of the practical activities. It would usually contain details and quantitative information, but these might be presented as an appendix if the project had a lot of results that could be better understood in a summarised form.
- Conclusions. This section is about what can be concluded from the results. If the project has been an investigation, it might present a view of the extent to which the questions addressed had been answered. If the project was carried out through a series of tasks and activities, this section would come to a conclusion about the extent to which the objectives of the project had been achieved. It might also return to the purpose of the project and comment on the extent to which the overall purpose had been achieved. The conclusions might also present some of the learning that has been gained during the project.

- Recommendations. This section will make recommendations that arise from the conclusions. For example, if the project failed to fully achieve an objective, a recommendation might be to pursue it in another way. If the purpose was not completely achieved, a recommendation might propose a way of achieving more. Recommendations might also propose the next steps necessary to progress the gains made by the project. If learning has been reported in the conclusions, these might give rise to recommendations as to how future benefits could be gained from doing things differently. Recommendations should always arise from the conclusions, which are, in turn, drawn from the previously presented results. This means that there will be a trail of evidence presented in a report that supports any further proposals made. Recommendations should be phrased as proposals for action and should be realistic and cautious. The action proposed will often be to investigate further and then to take action rather than trying to offer a sweeping solution to a problem.
- Acknowledgements, notes and references. These should acknowledge any contributions to the writing of the report, present any further notes indicated in the text and give full references for any quotations or references made in the text.
- Appendices. Anything essential to understanding of the report should be in the main text, but supplementary material or detailed data can be put into an appendix. Any material that would interrupt the flow of a report can also be put into an appendix. Nothing should be in an appendix that is not referred to in the report itself. It is not a dumping ground for anything that might be of interest to the reader. Details of budgets, statistics, personnel (usually only mentioned in confidential reports), relevant records, charts and diagrams are often included as appendices.

This is not an exhaustive list, but an indication of the structure that a report would normally follow. If the report is intended for a specific group or individual the structure will be similar to this, but the focus and content would reflect the particular interests of that audience. If the report is to be presented for academic assessment there would normally be additional sections, probably one reporting research carried out into the issues of the project and another presenting a critical review of the project.

Reports are often presented in numbered sections. There is no particular rule about how to number, but it is important to be consistent. The main sections are often numbered as 1, 2, 3, etc. with subsections being numbered as 1.1, 1.2, 1.3, etc. For a short report it is not always necessary to have subsections.

It is usual to be as brief as possible in a report while presenting the issues clearly. Try to avoid description unless it is essential for the point to be made. Read each sentence asking yourself why that sentence is there and what it adds. Read each paragraph and ask what point it makes and try to keep to one main point in each paragraph. Use bullet points, lists, diagrams and tables to help to present information concisely but clearly.

## REPORTING THE PROJECT TO GAIN AN ACADEMIC OR PROFESSIONAL AWARD

Projects and project reports are often included in programmes of learning when the students are working in management or professional positions and can carry out a project related to their work. There are a number of reasons for this.

### To link learning about theory and practice

It is often difficult to understand how theory applies in practical settings. Projects are often set as assignments in which a learner is usually asked

- to apply the theories and techniques introduced in a course to the setting in which he or she works;
- to make a critical appraisal of the extent to which each theory or technique was relevant and useful;
- to reflect on personal learning derived from carrying out the assignment.

### To consolidate learning

A project is often set as the final assignment for a course or section of a course, as it offers the opportunity to bring together many different aspects of learning and may contribute to useful consolidation and integration. Many educators think that it is important to put theory into practice if it is to be thoroughly understood.

### To provide evidence of learning for assessment

Projects are often used as evidence that a learner has achieved all of the intended learning outcomes of a course. Assessment can be carried out against the stated criteria and learning outcomes if the project is prepared so that all of the necessary evidence is presented.

## To enable the learner to make a useful workplace contribution related to their studies

Many learners who are sponsored by their organisations welcome the opportunity to carry out a project so that they can share the benefits of their studies. Employers usually welcome the use of projects in learning programmes and will normally offer their support and co-operation. In many programmes learners have a mentor from their organisation who will also help them to interpret the theories and techniques that they have learnt in terms of the issues in the workplace.

The key point about using a project as part of a programme of learning is that it is about applying course ideas in a practical setting. If your usual job makes it inappropriate for you to carry out a project at work there are two options that you might consider. You can negotiate to carry out a project in a different part of your organisation. People are often encouraged to do this if they are seeking a more senior position and need more evidence of leadership and management capability. Another possibility is to offer to carry out a project for another organisation, acting in a consultancy position. Many charities and voluntary organisations are glad to welcome people who look for this type of opportunity.

# MAKING EFFECTIVE PRESENTATIONS

Most people have some concerns about making presentations. Some people are quite fearful and try to avoid having to make a presentation. For someone in a leadership or management position, presentation is a skill that is important to learn and to practice because it will often be required.

There are many different types of presentation and their styles usually reflect the purpose and nature of the audience. It is often necessary to make a brief, informal presentation to a work group or team, and you may not even have thought of that as a presentation. If you have to organise your thoughts, put your ideas into some sort of order and then communicate them to others orally in a face-to-face setting, you are making a presentation. For a more formal presentation you may use visual aids and you may have to present your information and yourself in a more formal manner. It is this aspect of a presentation that can be rather frightening – we are not simply presenting something on paper that will carry its message without our physical presence. When we give a presentation we are part of the message that we send. Our appearance, manner, voice and gestures all contribute to the presentation. The response of the audience and the atmosphere created by the presentation influence the feelings of both presenter and audience. Because of our physical involvement, a presentation is a very personal event.

## ACTIVITY 16.1

*Allow 10 minutes.*

Identify the kinds of presentation that you have to make as part of your job. If you have not made any formal presentations, think about informal ones when you have been asked to give some information to colleagues.

Think back to a presentation that you have made that went really well and one that you feel could have been better. Using your recollections of those two presentations, identify your strengths and the areas where you need to improve.

You may have identified quite a range of presentations, such as meetings with staff and colleagues, departmental and inter-departmental committee and board meetings. Depending on your role, you may also have to make external presentations to colleagues in other organisations, or at conferences or public meetings. You may have to present information to people who have difficulty in understanding you.

Your presentations may be extremely formal, as at conferences, or relatively informal when, for example, you are informing staff about the implications of a new policy. Most of them are likely to have been planned, giving you time to prepare adequately, but there will always be occasions when you are called into a meeting at short notice and have to think on your feet.

Identifying your fears about making presentations and thinking carefully about your strengths and weaknesses are the first steps in learning how to make them more effective. You should now know the areas you need to concentrate on and practice. Always remember, however, that the quality of most presentations is determined by the work put in before you open your mouth. Preparation is vital.

# UNDERSTANDING YOUR AUDIENCE

We often fear that we will make fools of ourselves, forget what we were going to say or that the audience will not want to hear what we have to say. If you are gripped by fears of that sort, think back to times when you have been a member of an audience for a presentation. You may have noticed whether the presenter was smart and efficient or seemed vague and unfocused, but you were probably interested in what they had to say and made allowances for any mistakes or hesitant moments. We judge people who make presentations much as we would judge them in any other work setting. The focus is on the work issue at the heart of the session. Your role as presenter is to introduce the issue with as much information as is necessary to stimulate discussion. This often involves giving some information, explaining things and raising questions. All of these things are familiar to you from your normal work.

Sometimes we know the audience very well and can be confident about how we expect them to receive the messages we are planning to present. Often, however, the audience is unknown to us and this can be very frightening if we think of an audience as an impersonal and homogenous mass. If, instead, you think of an audience as a group of individuals, it is easier to picture the different types of reactions that your presentation might provoke.

The members of the audience are usually there because they are interested in the topic that you are presenting. If you focus on how to present the content in a clear and well structured way this will help you to make an effective presentation. An effective presentation is not one in which the audience is entertained, it is one where the message is clearly communicated and understood. It is not necessary to try to be amusing and it can be embarrassing if jokes fall flat. Humour is difficult to manage in a presentation where you know very little about the audience because so many jokes are derived from differences of one type or another. It is safer to focus on the content of the presentation and to aim to communicate the key messages as clearly and appropriately as possible.

The key to an effective presentation is to match the purpose of your presentation with the particular members of the audience in a way that will help them to understand the message you are sending. It is important to pitch the presentation at a level that will be understandable and to use appropriate language. It is very helpful in planning your presentation to find out as much as you can about the audience before you decide exactly how to make your presentation. Ask yourself the following questions and try to find out anything that you don't know.

A crucial part of your preparation should be to consider the audience and what they will be wanting from your presentation.

- How many people will be there?
- Who are they and what are their roles?
- Do you know any of them?
- Will they know who you are and why you're there?
- How will they expect you to appear?
- What are they expecting from your presentation? (Be realistic.)
- What do you want to achieve? (Are you aiming to inform or persuade?)
- Could you discuss what you want to say with some of the people who will be there before you finalise your presentation?

- How interested will your audience be in the subject?
- What level of knowledge will they have about it?
- Will they be familiar with any technical language or jargon? If not, you must either explain it or avoid using it.
- What levels of experience are they likely to have?
- Will they have any preconceptions or misconceptions of the subject? If so, how will you deal with that?
- How are they likely to respond to the presentation? Remember that you want to achieve your purpose.
- Do they respect your knowledge, experience and opinions?
- Might what you have to say be controversial?
- How might they use what you have to say?

The answers to these questions are important in helping you to make your preparations. Once you have found out about your audience and their expectations, you will have a realistic idea of what you need to offer them in the presentation. You can then move on to planning your presentation. It is essential to give yourself enough time to prepare well, so don't leave everything to the last minute. Inadequate planning and preparation are the cause of most poor presentations.

## PURPOSE AND CONTENT

Start your preparation by thinking carefully about the following questions.

- What is the main purpose of your presentation?
- What do you want your audience to do as a result of your presentation?
- What is the overall message you want to deliver?
- What are the main points you need to make to get your message across?
- What supporting information are you likely to need and where can you obtain it?
- What would be the most informative and interesting title for your presentation?
- How much time do you have? Will this include time for questions?
- Would it be helpful to give the audience any information in advance, such as statistics you will use to illustrate or support your case?
- Would visual aids, such as overhead projector transparencies, clarify important points and aid understanding?
- How can you best anticipate and prepare for the questions that you may be asked?
- Have you been asked to bring copies of your paper or summaries for distribution after the presentation, or would it be helpful to do so?

## STRUCTURE

Once you have clarified who your audience will be, what you want to achieve and what you need to cover, you can begin to plan the structure of your talk. Most presentations use the following general structure:

- introduction – what you will cover in the presentation and whether you will take questions as you go or at the end;
- middle – the main points you want to make and the evidence to support those points;
- end – conclusions, recommendations and summary of what has been covered.

The traditional *aide-mémoire* for making a presentation is:

- tell them what you're going to say;
- say it;
- tell them what you've said.

This is simplistic, but a good summary of what is important.

Use the following guidelines to help you to plan the structure and content:

- How can you match your purpose to the audience? (How can you best use your knowledge of your audience to decide what to include and the level to pitch it?)
- What is the most logical sequence for your presentation? (What key points do you want to make in your introduction, middle and conclusion?)
- How can you lead into your presentation to gain your audience's immediate attention? For example:
  - acknowledging their specific interests
  - beginning with an anecdote
  - outlining what you hope the audience will get from the presentation
  - asking a rhetorical question
  - explaining why you were invited to make the presentation.
- What information or data can you use to support your argument? (Don't try to cram everything you know on the subject into your talk. Select the main points, and include only as much detail as your audience will require or be able to absorb.)
- How can you relate your main points to each other to produce a cohesive argument?
- Where is it most appropriate to summarise to aid the flow of your presentation?
- What visual aids could you use to illustrate your points?
- What would be the most effective way to conclude your presentation?

You might now be thinking that this is an awful lot of work to do in planning the presentation, but if you do make thorough plans you are most of the way to ensuring that the presentation is effective.

## DELIVERY

There is no reason why you shouldn't play to your strongest qualities.

It is important to choose an approach to delivery that feels natural and comfortable. If you are comfortable with speaking to an audience, then all you need to do is to make sure that you don't wander away from the point so that you keep to time and deliver a purposeful presentation. If you are nervous about speaking to the audience, it is important to prepare ways that will help you to feel more comfortable.

One of the normal fears is that you will forget what you intended to say. It is not usually successful to write yourself a script and to read from it. The words and rhythms of speech are different from those of a written text. Your audience will expect eye contact and you can easily lose your place in a script and make yourself even more nervous. Speakers are usually more engaging if they talk as though they know about the issue and are enthusiastic about it.

A number of aids can help you to keep track of the sequence and key points:

- You can write the sequence of a talk on a card or sheet of paper so that you can refer to it if you need to. Write large and make sure you can see it clearly.
- Some people write the key points and a bit about them on small filing cards and hold them in their hands during the presentation. There is a danger of dropping them, but you can punch holes in the corners and use a treasury tag to hold them together so that you can fold them over as you use each.
- You can use overhead transparencies or Powerpoint screens to write the key points and they will also act as a reminder as you work through the talk.
- You can have notes with you in a form in which you can easily find the right place; tell the audience what you are doing if you find that you need to refer to them during the talk.

It is always very helpful to practise the talk beforehand, even if you feel very confident. You can find that you have misjudged the timing and need to speed up or slow down. Sometimes you may find that it is very hard to say a word or phrase that is important and you can either practise it or substitute the difficult section with something that is easier to handle.

Consider what your options are about where you stand and whether you would feel better leaning on something or even sitting down. If you are very nervous, it is often an option to sit and to focus the audience on the visual aid rather than on yourself. If you use an overhead projector or make a computer-based presentation you will probably want to darken the room, so check that you will still be able to see your notes if you are using them. Check any electrical equipment before the audience arrive if you possibly can. Make sure that you are confident about how to turn it on and use it.

Usually, presenters have to introduce themselves and explain the purpose of the presentation. Focus on ensuring that the audience is comfortable and ready to listen to you and remember that your job is to convey the message clearly. Some guidelines are:

- Project your voice to the furthest member of the group. If unsure, ask if they can hear.
- Act enthusiastically, make and maintain eye contact, smile, try to look relaxed and to make your introduction without looking at your notes.
- Act confidently and your audience will believe that you are confident.
- Speak clearly and at conversational speed. Don't mumble, rush your words or use a monotone delivery. Use the natural inflections of conversation.
- Control your audience by maintaining eye contact and by looking for and responding to signs of puzzlement or boredom.
- Avoid distracting your audience with unnecessary pacing around, fiddling or gesturing.
- Make sure that you keep an eye on the time. Having to rush through the last few points will mean that you won't do justice to your argument.
- Lead up to your concluding remarks by signposting the way. Phrases such as 'And my final point is' or 'If I can just sum up my main points' will let your audience know that the end is in sight so they can expect some conclusions and recommendations or a summary.
- Finish as enthusiastically as you began. Make sure that your audience has got the message you wanted to deliver and finish on a high point.
- Think about what questions might be asked and how you will reply.

The only way to become confident and competent in making presentations is to practise, to listen to feedback and to try to do a little better each time. To develop your skills you will need to ensure that you have some opportunities to make presentations if these have not previously been a natural part of your job. As with most skills, the key to improving your performance is self-evaluation and practice. Try to get into the habit of taking a few minutes after each presentation to assess what has gone well and identify any lessons for the future. In addition, whenever you listen to other people's presentations, note any features that made them particularly interesting and informative or, conversely, ineffective.

CHAPTER 17

# LEARNING FROM THE PROJECT

An organisation can benefit from each project by trying to learn how future projects can be more efficient and effective. It is also possible to learn how people in the organisation can share what is learnt more widely so that good practice can be identified and adopted in other appropriate areas of work.

The nature of a project as separate from day-to-day work makes it possible for the skills, experience and understanding necessary to be successful in a particular project role to be identified. It is also possible for people to take roles in projects that are different from their normal roles at work. Projects can often provide a training ground for teamworking and leadership while delivering the project objectives.

Different types of learning for individuals and for organisations can be gained from a project. For this learning to be useful, it needs to be recognised and captured so that it can inform future development.

## ORGANISATIONAL LEARNING ABOUT MANAGEMENT OF PROJECTS

Organisational learning is a difficult concept because organisations vary considerably and learning is an intangible process. If the word 'learning' is used in its widest sense, it is essential to development and maturity. If an organisation is not able to learn, it is unable to develop and may soon fail to succeed in a fast-changing world.

Learning can be identified and noted at any stage of a project if people are aware of the potential to learn and willing to share that learning more widely. It is often convenient to hold a review of each stage of a project. The stage might not have completed any project deliverables, but progress can be reviewed alongside consideration of what could have been done better and what barriers to progress were encountered.

It can be helpful to hold a final structured debriefing process, to include stakeholders as well as all the members of the project team.

This may take the form of a series of meetings to draw conclusions about overall project performance. Any constraints encountered would be considered and proposals for overcoming them in future projects noted. It is important to identify and review any new ways of working that were developed and to consider what was effective and what could have been done differently.

A formal system can also be used to ensure that individuals with key responsibilities are debriefed when their tasks or activities are completed. Individual interviews can be held with key members of the project team, for example the managers of key stages or leaders of specialist tasks. Interviewers can encourage people to evaluate their performance and identify what they have learnt from the experience personally, but also to identify what lessons could be learnt by the organisation.

Learning areas for organisations are often about the ways in which projects fit into the normal structures and procedures and the extent to which these help or hinder the use of project working to achieve focused outcomes. There is often tension in running a project in an organisation that is not structured to carry out most or all of its work through project working, because staff are often expected to be managed and to behave in two different ways.

One area of learning to consider is that of how to structure project working within the organisational environment in a way that enables the project to benefit from the full potential of the project team. This may involve releasing staff from their day-to-day work entirely, maybe by funding temporary replacements, or by partially replacing staff for the duration of the project but lengthening the time-scale of the project to enable it to be completed by a part-time project team. Another solution might be to employ staff purely for the duration of the project on fixed-term contracts. This may solve the staffing problem, but may make it difficult to incorporate outcomes from the project to change or develop the organisation because the permanent staff may feel that the project and its aims have nothing to do with them and that their ideas have not been wanted.

**Example 17.1 – Lessons for the organisation from a project**

The project manager of a project that had required considerable staff training identified a number of lessons learned from the project. She listed these in the final project report:

- Ensure that the project leader's role and accountabilities are clearly understood at an early stage.
- Make a detailed estimate of the staff resources to show how the normal work of staff transferred to the project will be covered.

- Replacement costs for staff sent on training courses should be included in the budget.
- Project planning and implementation are not sequential – plans have to be flexible.
- The objectives of the project need to be clear.
- Plan communications and do not assume that networks already exist.
- Make involvement of key individuals in development activities mandatory – we must be open to change and influential people can block it if they are not supportive.
- Manage the tension between operational work and project development work.

The report was received with interest and the project manager was asked to run a workshop for senior staff to help them to decide how to make use of the lessons she had identified. In the workshop they considered the conditions from which the lessons had been drawn and spent time in agreeing how to avoid these and similar pitfalls in future project working.

One of the problems with identifying learning from a project is that learning is often derived from experience of things going wrong. People often don't want to say much about what has gone wrong, particularly in an organisation that tends to focus on blaming and punishing. Senior staff can help to encourage a climate in which learning is shared by ensuring that people are treated fairly when mistakes are made and that responsibility is shared for repairing any damage and for making sure that lessons are learnt.

Organisations that use projects frequently often develop formal procedures to guide those leading and managing their projects. Some also create resources in the forms of guidelines and examples to help their staff to write project proposals and to prepare the documentation that is needed throughout the project.

## SHARING LEARNING FROM A PROJECT

One of the questions that concerns many of those responsible for developing staff in organisations is how the good practice of one team can be shared to improve others. There are a number of ways of trying to do this:

- Create a database. Written information provides a way of storing the ideas, but it is going to be useful only if people seek it out and read it. It may not be easy to understand unless those reading the information already know a lot about the issues and the normal practice in that area of work.

- Give a demonstration. This can be a much more engaging and direct way of showing how something can be done differently than simply offering a written description. Many of the details shown in a demonstration can be illuminating and the ideas may be conveyed immediately to people who already carry out similar work. A demonstration is unlikely to be enough to equip someone to carry out a new procedure unless they already have considerable knowledge and skill.
- Visit and enquire. Where there is one successful team other teams can visit them to watch them in action and to question them as their visitors for a short time. This can be more helpful than a demonstration because people can check out their understanding and ask questions. It is also often very helpful to see a skilled performance in the setting in which it works well.
- Coach and supervise. These are more long-term approaches that involve working closely with each other so that the one who is learning can try out the new way of working with the help and support of the more experienced person. If one team is teaching another these roles can still be effective, sometimes with people in each team pairing up and also with the whole teaching team working with the whole learning team.

When projects have been successful because of the ways in which the team worked, or when a project is about changing working practices, these approaches to transferring learning can be considered as possible ways of disseminating the learning that has been gained.

## INDIVIDUAL DEVELOPMENT FROM A PROJECT

For some staff, the invitation to take part in a project is welcomed as an opportunity for self-development. The development possible in a project includes gaining experience of contributing expertise in a different context, learning to do something different and gaining experience of acting in a role that is different. All of these are potentially valuable experiences as they can enhance a person's potential to be employed in a different capacity or to be promoted. A project manager can often support individuals who are seeking development through the project, but must always also consider the cost of doing that.

In some organisations project working is seen as an opportunity for staff development and projects are planned to include an appropriate mix of experienced and inexperienced staff and the resources to train and support where necessary. In others, inexperienced people in project teams can find themselves lost and unsupported, potentially becoming a burden on the project. In some ways, projects are like a small organisation and can plan for staff development in a similar way. Ideally, staff are appointed to the project team because they have the appropriate mix of skills, knowledge and experience. In practice, this is often not possible because of time-scales and staff availability.

If staff are willing but need some training and support, a project manager can often arrange for coaching and supervision within the resources of the project. If a member of staff can be helped to become productive quickly, this is often a pragmatic approach if more experienced staff are willing to take on a training role. These staff can also gain from taking on a new role, as they can be supported as coaches and supervisors and gain experience and credit for that aspect of their work. Similarly, more experienced staff may agree to mentor staff taking leadership, management or expert roles for the first time. The mentors may not be on the project team but would need to understand the demands of the roles involved.

Sometimes more formal training is needed. If this can be provided quickly, for example training to use a new computer package, it may be appropriate to provide it. There is a problem, however, when training is unlikely to lead to an effective performance within the time-scales needed to complete the activities of the project. If this is the case, it may be better to accept that the appointment was a mistake and take steps to make a new appointment.

## MANAGEMENT DEVELOPMENT THROUGH LEADING A PROJECT

There is an opportunity to use the experience of managing a project to develop yourself for a more senior role and to demonstrate from the successful outcomes and evaluation of the project that you are prepared for such a role.

For many managers, taking responsibility for a project provides a time-bounded task with clear objectives and a fixed budget. A project usually involves managing across a wide range of areas that are normally managed in separate departments. It usually includes management of staff, finance, operations and information. It often involves managing complicated interactions and difficult situations. There is usually a strategic dimension in ensuring that the project continues to align with organisational objectives and directions. Because of this variety, a project can provide a boundaried world within an organisation that is similar to the view that a senior manager or director must take of a whole organisation.

**Example 17.2 – Personal learning in a project**

A person who was managing a project for the first time made this list of personal learning objectives:

- To improve planning, controlling and negotiating skills. I'll know if I've done this by keeping a record of all occasions when I use these skills and each outcome.

- To learn skills in developing a team. I'll keep a note of the things I do to help the team to develop and of things that go particularly well or not very well. I'll try to note the impact I have each time I intervene.
- To improve skills in resource management (human and financial). This is the first time that I'll have held a budget and I want to make good use of it. I've arranged to have regular meetings with our finance officer. I'm also worried about overseeing all the HR issues and I've arranged to meet the personnel officer to make sure that I understand all the responsibilities that I should take on with this project.
- To improve skills in collection and interpretation of data. I have some experience with figures and with statistics, but I'm not very sure that I understand qualitiative data. I'm planning to discuss this with my mentor.
- To develop confidence in leading change. This is another one that I'll want to work on with my mentor. I'm sure that I can handle the planning but the implementation will be new for me.
- To involve service users. My role has not been directly with service users in the past, but I'm sure that they should be consulted about this project. I shall plan the consultation with others in the team and shall take a lead in the meetings or workshops we decide to hold.

All of these objectives will be completed during the period of the project. I will review all of the objectives regularly with my mentor.

You might consider carrying out a personal self-evaluation to plan your development during the period in which you carry out the role of project manager. Some of the information you will need might be obtained from your last appraisal and you might already have a personal development plan. If you are to be successful as a project manager you will need skills in:

- planning;
- managing routines and systems;
- organising to achieve outcomes within constraints;
- negotiating;
- motivating and influencing people;
- communications;
- managing the big picture and the detail;
- maintaining progress and overcoming obstacles;
- decision making;
- diplomacy;
- managing emotions;
- managing information;
- handling interpersonal relationships.

This list is not exhaustive, but could provide the basis for an analysis of the extent to which you have development needs in any of these areas.

## ACTIVITY 17.1

*Allow 10 minutes.*

Imagine that you have just been asked to manage a new project that will be more challenging than any that you have managed before. Make a note of any ways in which you might plan for personal development and how you would then evaluate the development that you had achieved.

There are a number of areas in which you might have considered planning personal development. The broad areas might include improving your skills in managing a project, your knowledge of techniques in managing projects and your understanding of the process of managing a project. In particular, you might have noted skills areas including interpersonal relationships, leadership, effective communications, management of control systems, management of relationships with partners and stakeholders. You might have focused on developing your understanding of techniques by applying new knowledge in a new situation.

Evaluation of personal development can be carried out using approaches similar to those you would use to evaluate other things. First, you need to set targets or criteria so that you can assess whether you have achieved the development that you intend. Ask yourself, 'How shall I know that I have succeeded?' and identify the most significant indicators. As the project proceeds, you can collect evidence relating to your personal achievements in the same way as you would collect evidence relating to the project objectives. You may choose to do this by compiling a portfolio of evidence to demonstrate your achievements against each objective that you have set yourself. Another way to keep a record would be by keeping a project journal in which to make notes, to keep other evidence and to keep a record of what you notice and learn as the project develops. Some people find it very helpful to note what works better than they expected and what works less well than expected and to look for reasons for this. It is sometimes possible to identify underlying causes of both success and failure by keeping a personal record of this nature.

---

It can be lonely managing a project and it can be difficult to seek feedback about your own performance if the team is new and its members lack confidence or if the situation requires you to take a strong lead. Consider asking a senior manager in your organisation to act as a mentor to you for the duration of the project. This should not be someone who is a direct stakeholder in the project, but someone who can help you to learn from what happens as the process unfolds, without having a strong personal stake in any of the project outcomes. Share with your mentor your plans to use the project for personal development and ask them to help you to scope out the opportunities the project offers.

You might find that it is helpful to use the framework of a personal development plan, indicating some targets for development and identifying how you will know that you have succeeded. You might also want to collect evidence of your achievements to support your claims as you consider new career options.

# RECOMMENDED FURTHER READING

## For more about being a manager in health and care settings

*Managing in Health and Social Care* by Vivien Martin and Euan Henderson, 2001, co-published by the Open University and Routledge.

This book was based on the learning materials prepared by the Open University Business School, in partnership with the Department of Health and the Institute for Healthcare Management, for the Management Education Scheme by Open Learning (MESOL). Anyone with little management experience will find sections in this book to help them with the general management tasks that are needed throughout the management of any project. In particular, there are chapters on improving your effectiveness, working with values and vision, managing change, finding out what service users want, management styles, motivation, leading and teamworking, working with standards, working with a budget and planning an investigation.

## For a broader understanding of managing in complex situations

*Understanding Organisations* by Charles Handy, 1999 (4th edition with a new introduction), published by Penguin Books.

This is a 'classic' book that introduces many of the key concepts and ideas that are found in foundation management courses. There are strong links between practice and theory, with many examples and illustrations. The areas that are covered include motivation, roles and interactions in organisations, leadership, power and influence, group working and organisational culture. This book also offers many helpful suggestions for the further study of management.

## For information about some of the best-known management theories and ideas

*Writers on Organizations* by Derek S. Pugh and David J. Hickson, 1996 (5th edition), published by Penguin Books.

This book is for those who would like to know more of the most influential ideas about how organisations work and where these ideas have come from. The book sets out many well-known theories, explaining how the ideas developed and how they have been applied.

## For more information about managing large projects

*Project Management* by Mike Field and Laurie Keller, 1998, co-published by the Open University and International Thomson Business Press.

This book is written in the form of learning materials and is intended for people managing projects in any type of organisation. It pays particular attention to the issues relating to industrial and technological projects and would be helpful for anyone managing a long or complex project in those areas. It deals in more detail with some of the complexities of planning and scheduling.

## For practical help in planning your own management development

*Develop your Management Potential* by John Coopey and John Beech with Charlotte Chambers and Adrian McLean, 1993 (second edition), London: Kogan Page.

This book is a self-help guide to management development. It helps you to review your management experience and to identify areas for development. The book is designed to be used quite flexibly. There is a section dealing with ways of planning development at work and another on choosing more formal development programmes that lead to qualifications.

# INDEX